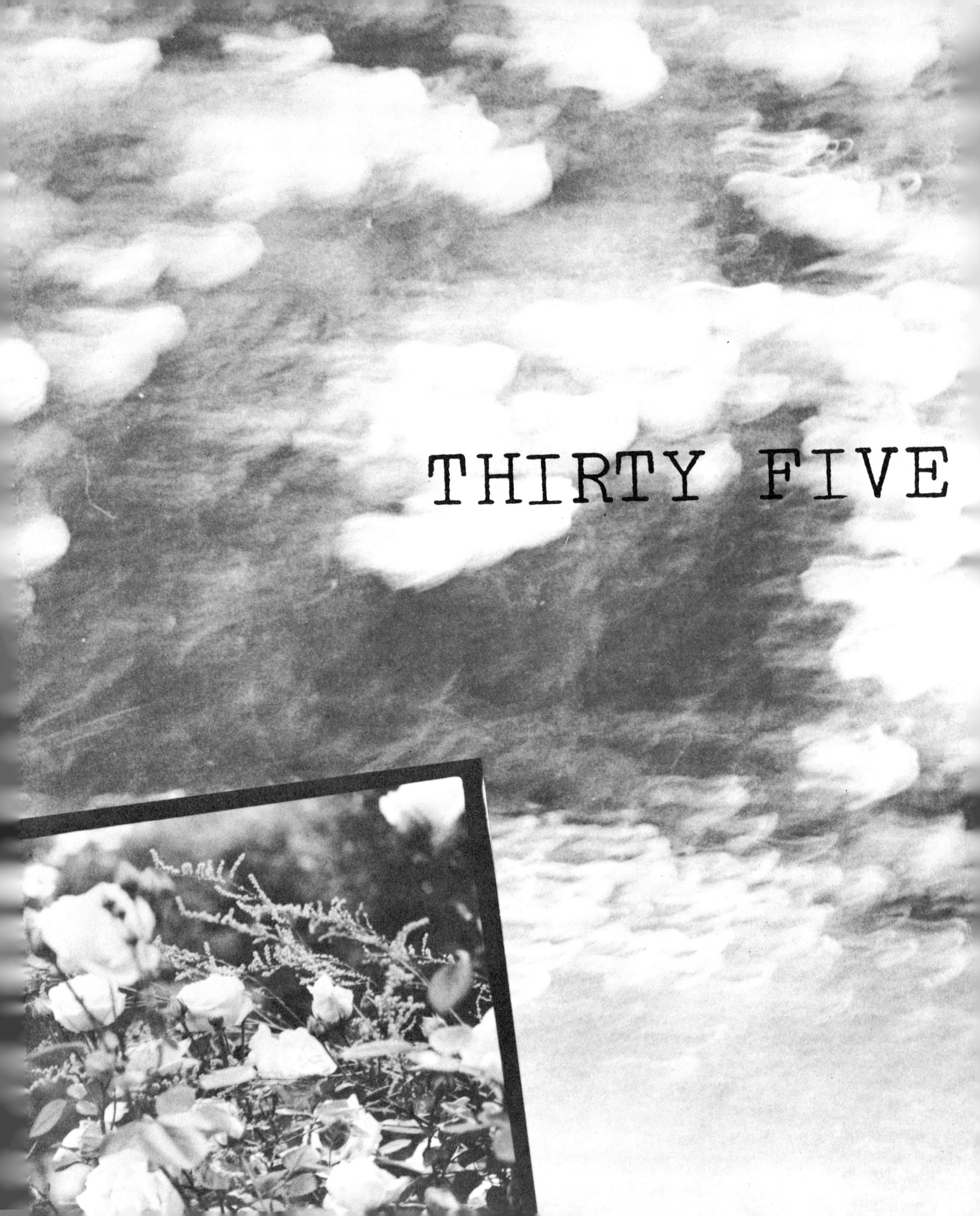
THIRTY FIVE

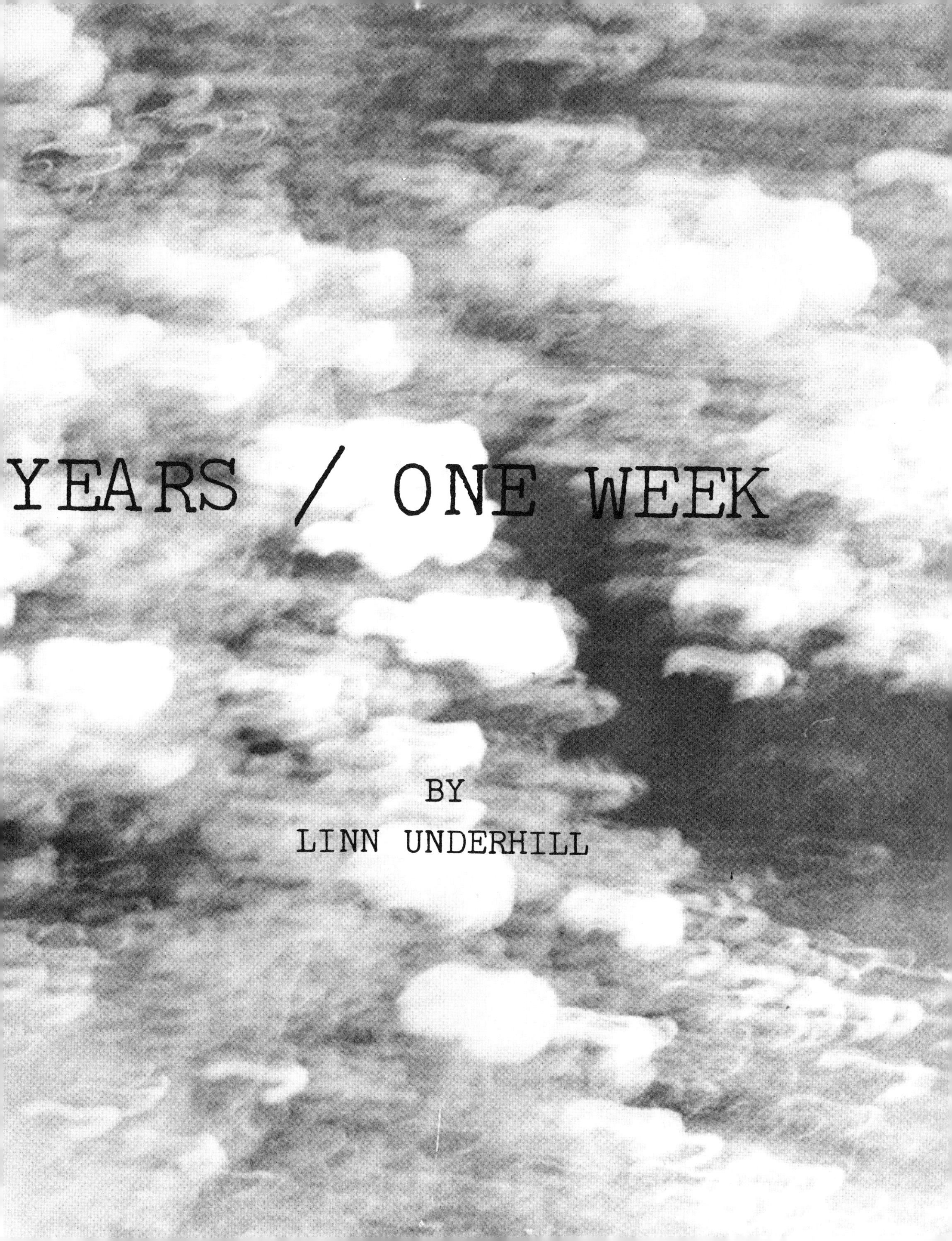

YEARS / ONE WEEK

BY

LINN UNDERHILL

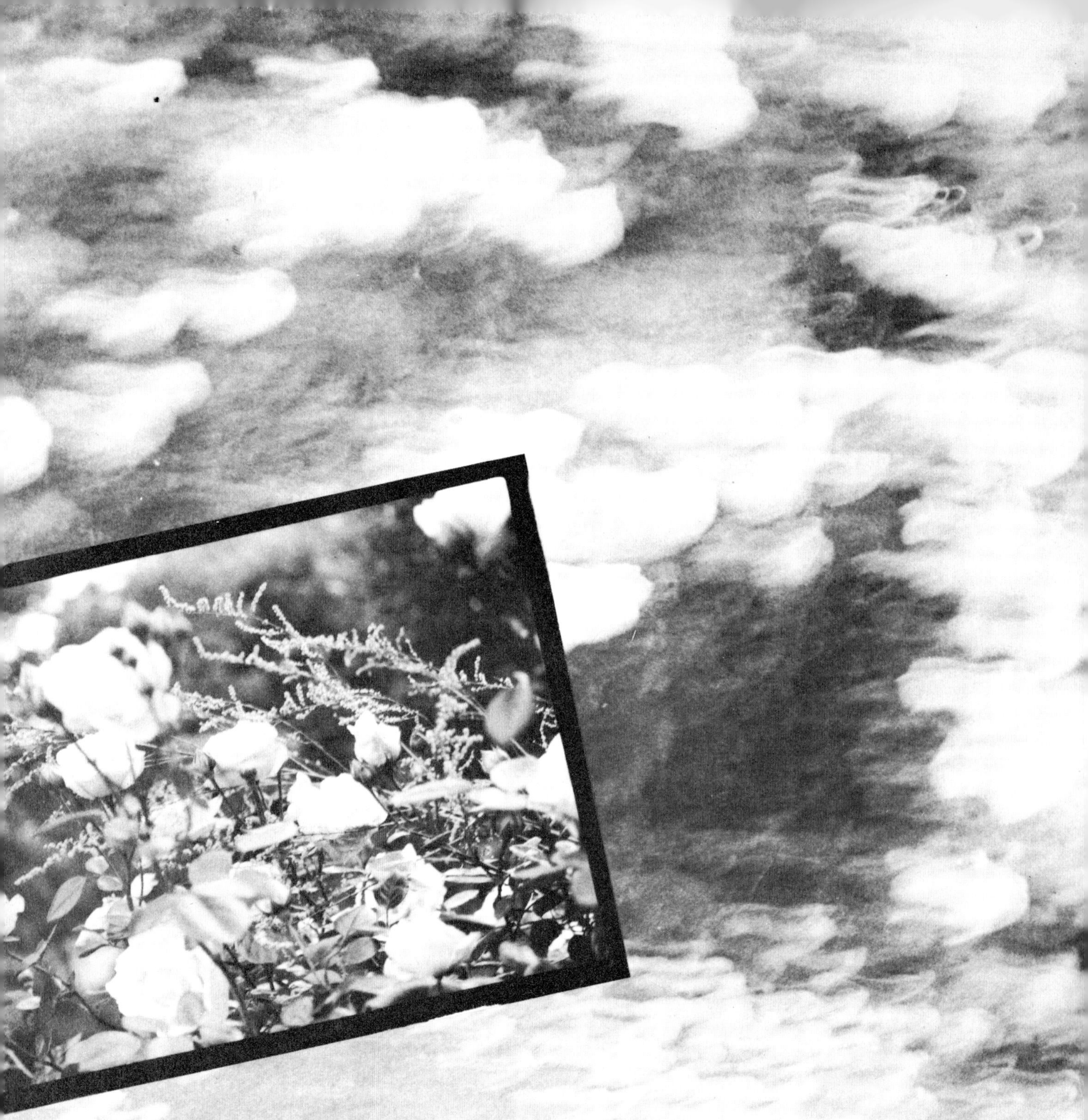

VISUAL STUDIES WORKSHOP PRESS
31 PRINCE STREET, ROCHESTER, NEW YORK 14607

LC CATALOG CARD NO. 81-070286
ISBN 0-89822-019-X

THIS BOOK WAS SUPPORTED BY AN INDIVIDUAL PROJECTS GRANT
FROM THE NEW YORK STATE COUNCIL ON THE ARTS.

IN MEMORY OF MY YOUNGER SISTER
BEVERLY BALDWIN KAHN
"CHER"

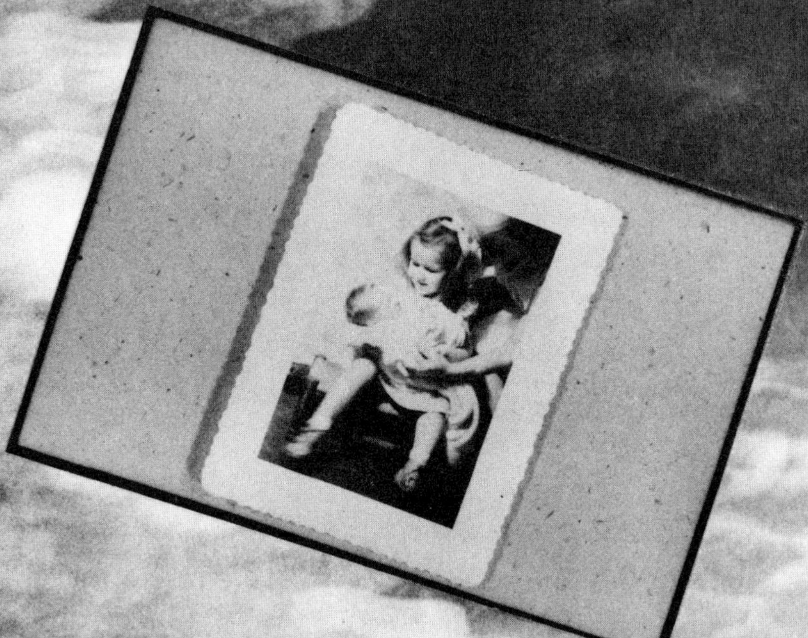

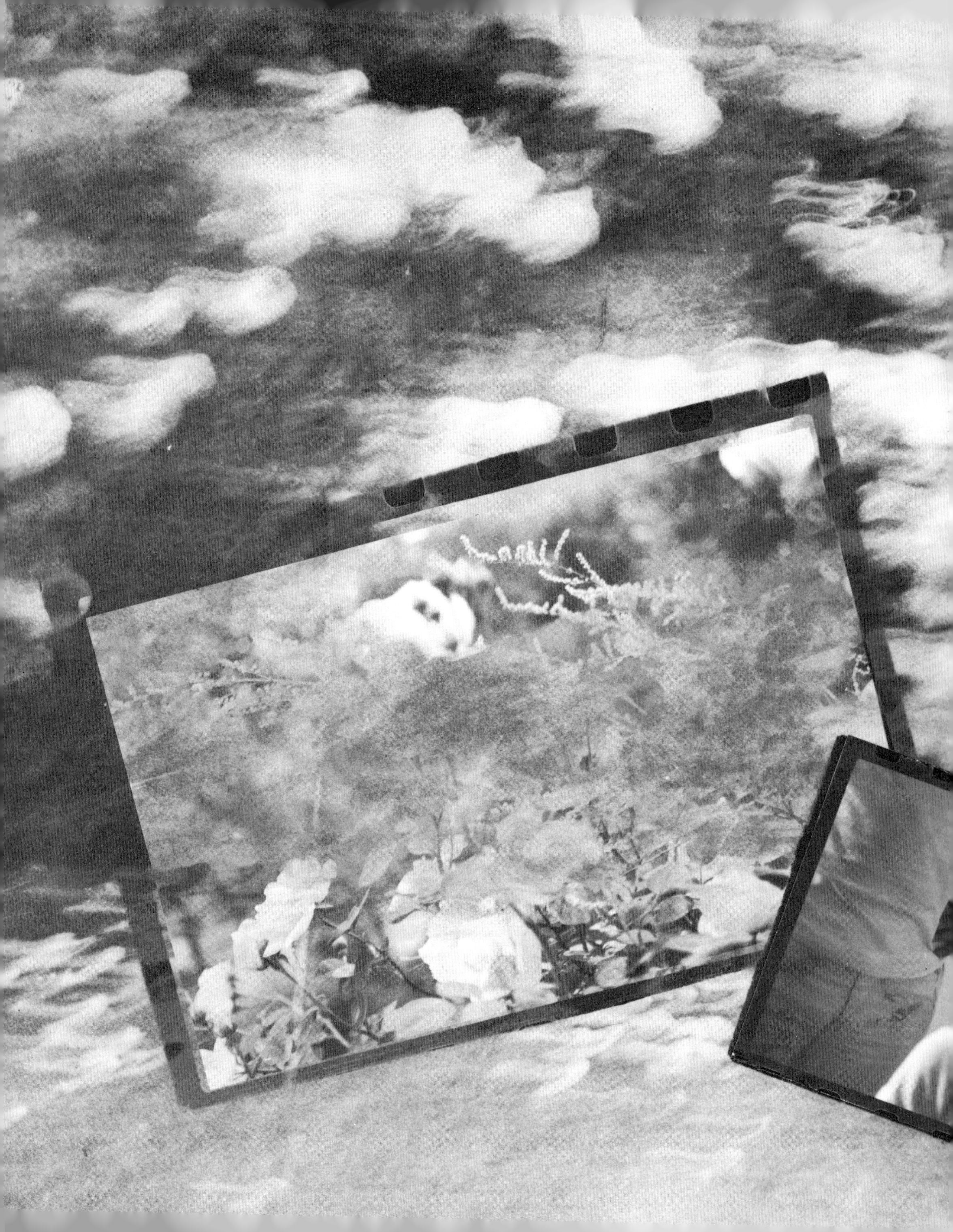

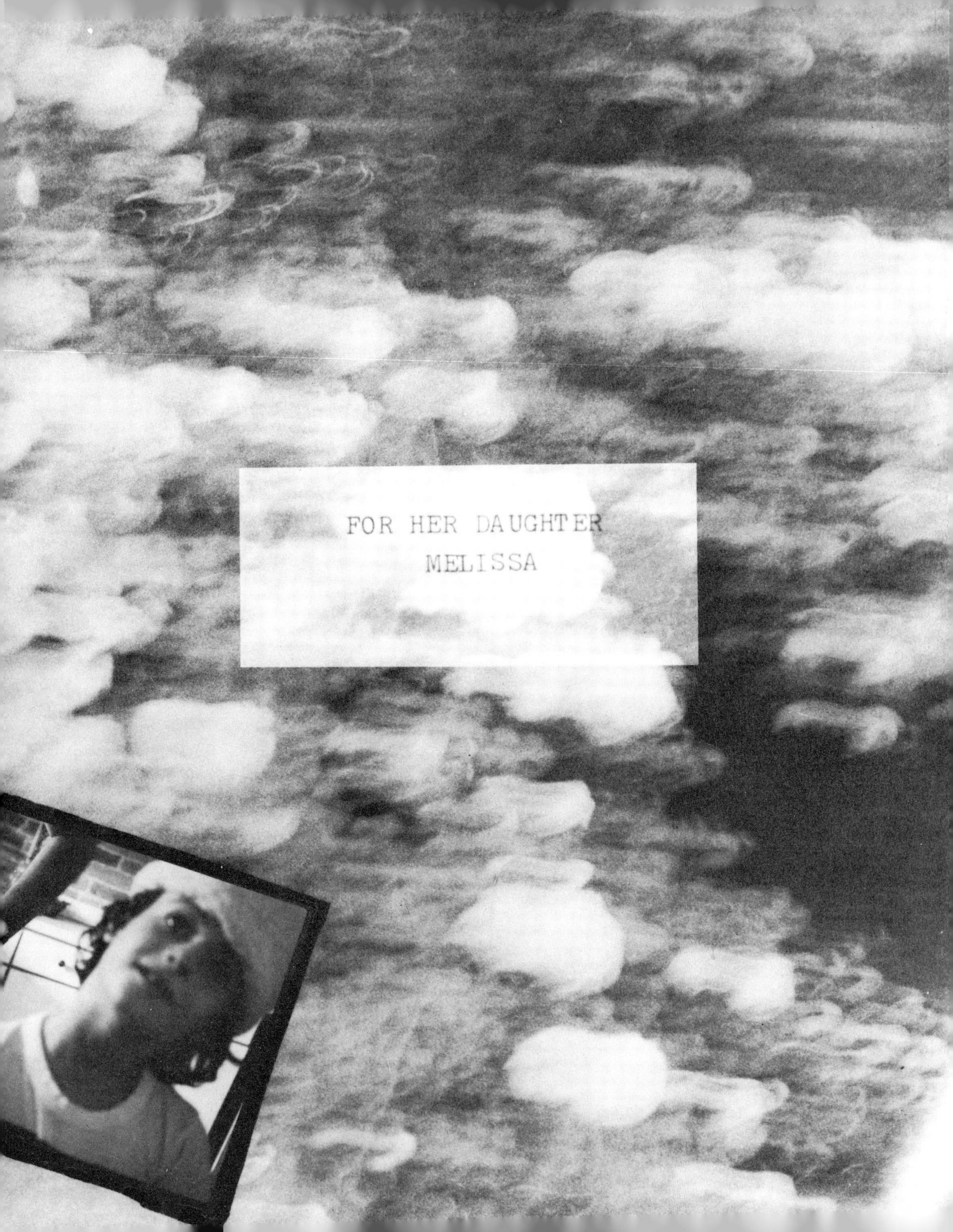
FOR HER DAUGHTER
MELISSA

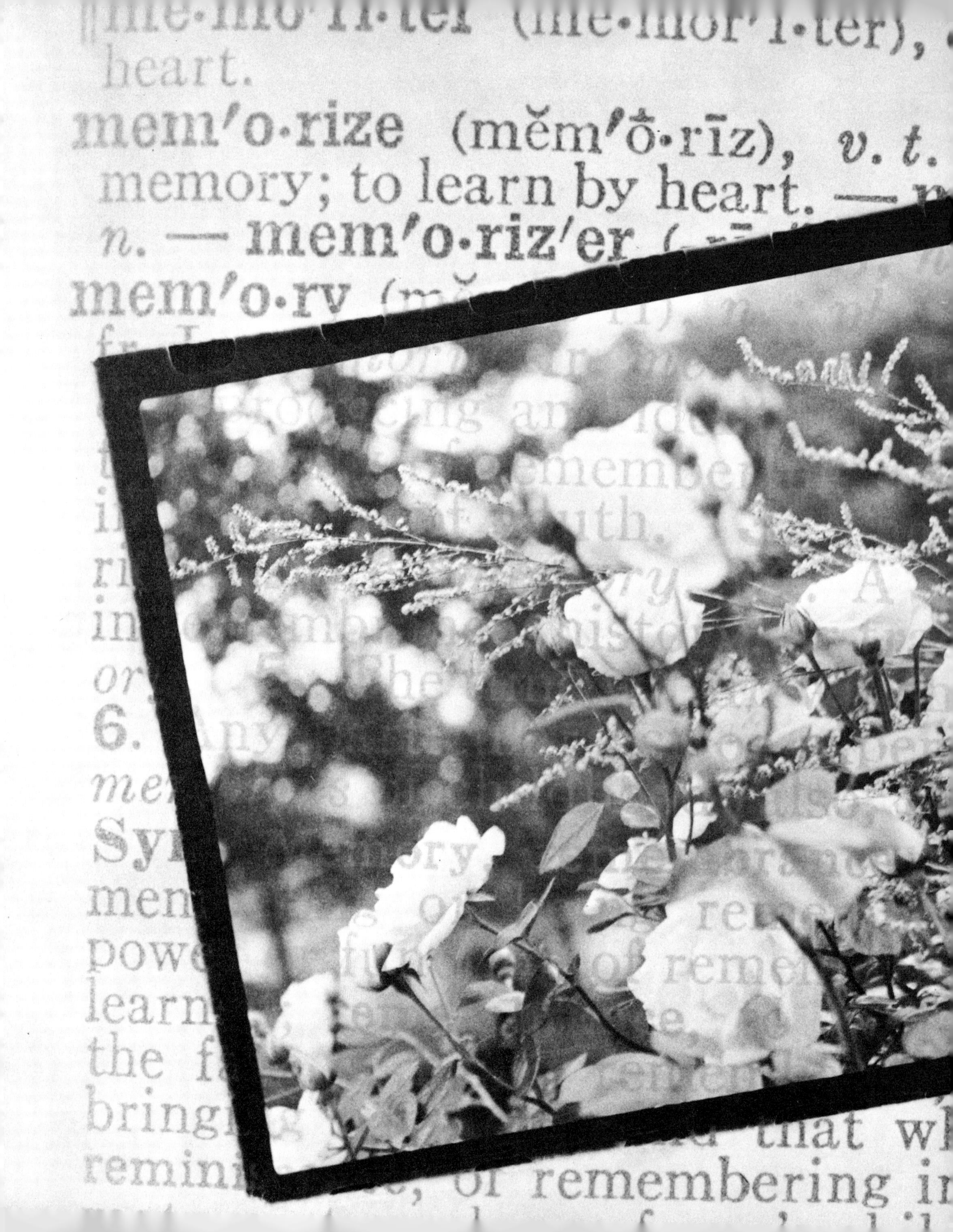
heart.
mem'o·rize (mĕm'ō·rīz), v. t.
memory; to learn by heart.
n. — mem'o·riz'er
mem'o·ry
reminiscence, or remembering i

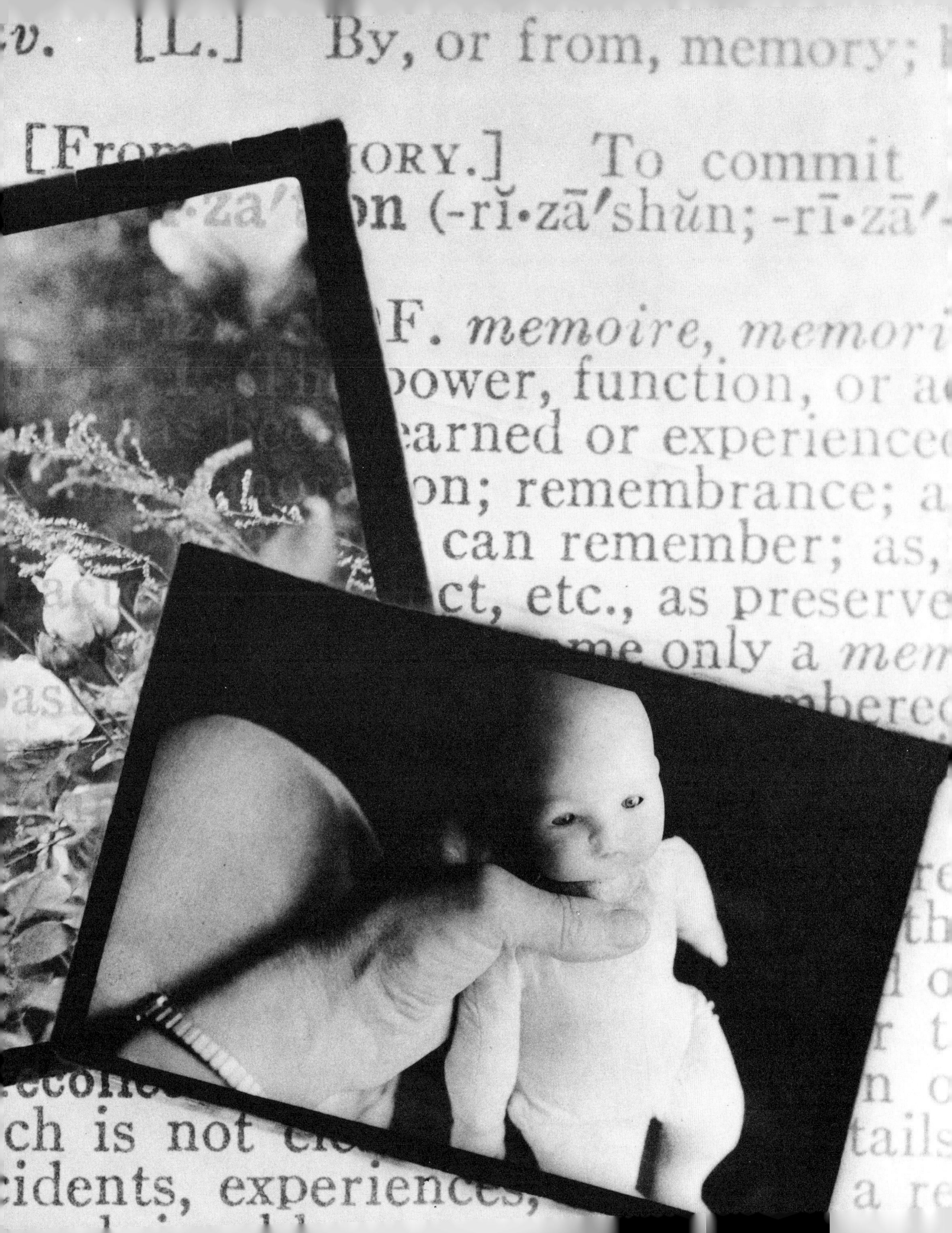
By, or from, memory;
To commit
F. memoire,
power, function, or
earned or experience
remembrance;
can remember; as,
etc., as preserve
only a
ch is not
cidents, experiences,

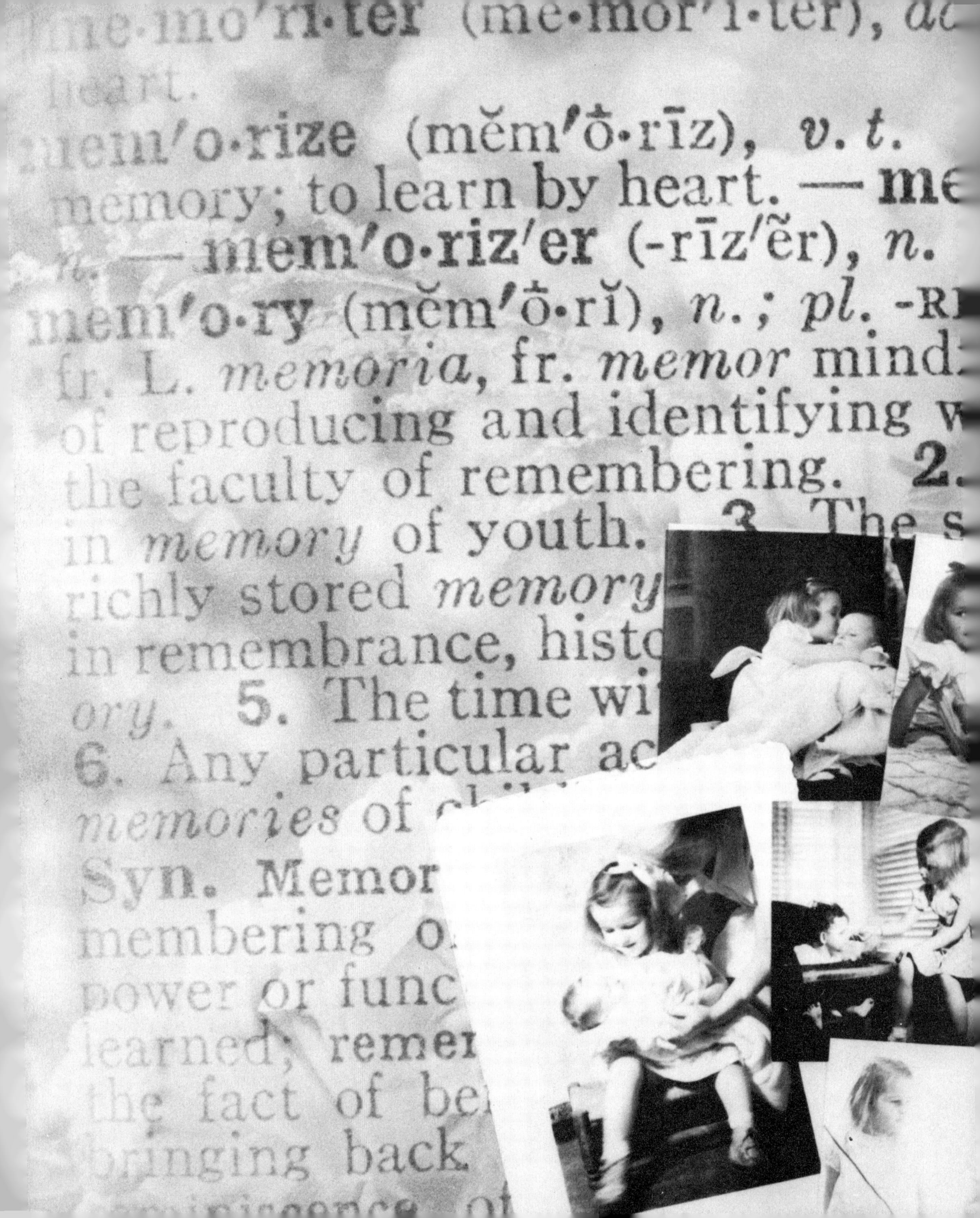
mem'o·rize (mĕm'ō·rīz), v. t.
memory; to learn by heart. — me
— mem'o·riz'er (-rīz'ẽr), n.
mem'o·ry (mĕm'ō·rĭ), n.; pl. -R
fr. L. memoria, fr. memor mind
of reproducing and identifying w
the faculty of remembering. 2.
in memory of youth.
richly stored memory
in remembrance, histo
ory. 5. The time wi
6. Any particular ac
memories of
Syn. Memor
membering o
power or func
learned; remem
the fact of be
bringing back

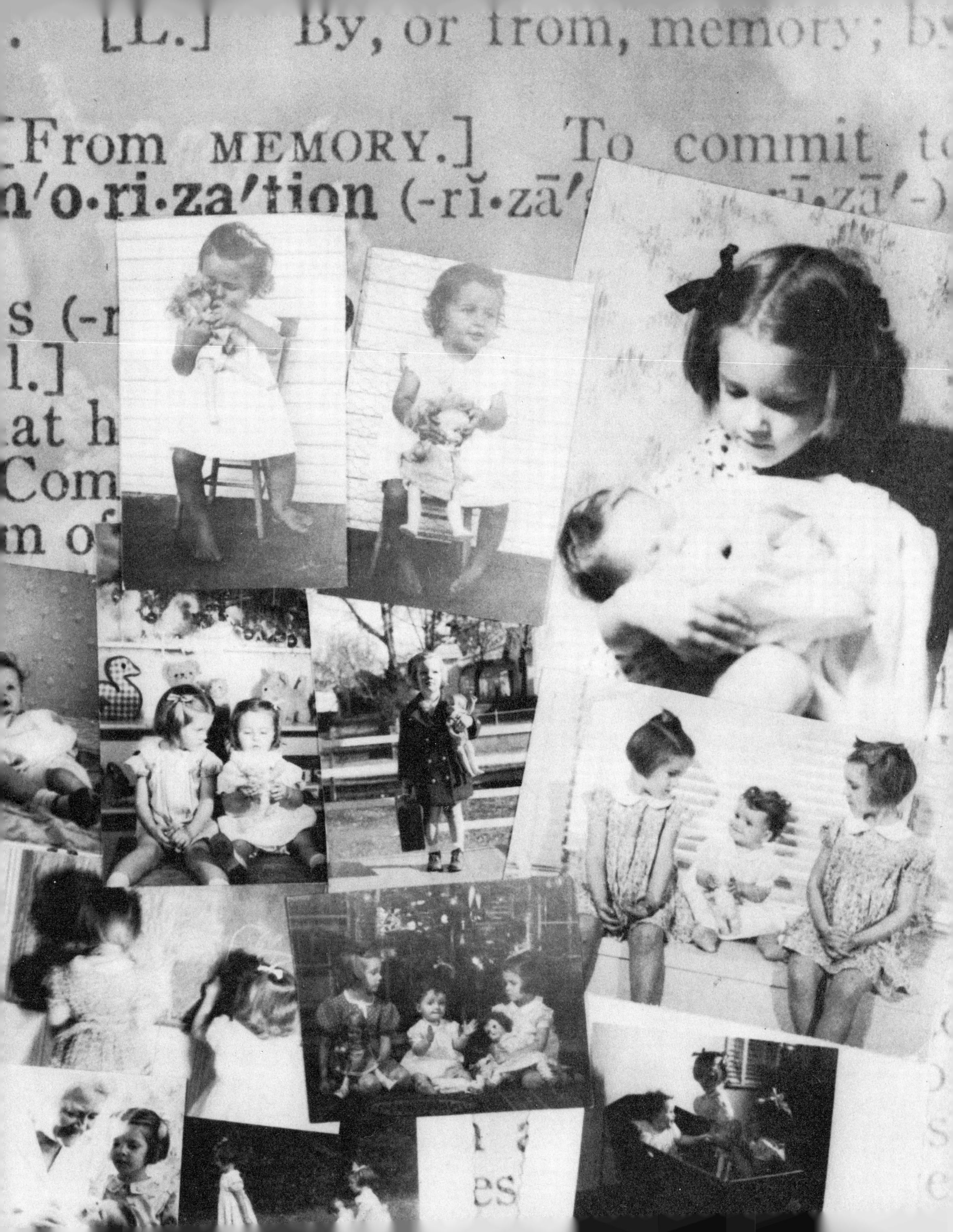
[L.] By, or from, memory; by
[From MEMORY.] To commit t
n'o·ri·za'tion (-rĭ·zā'
s (-r
l.]
at h
Com
n o

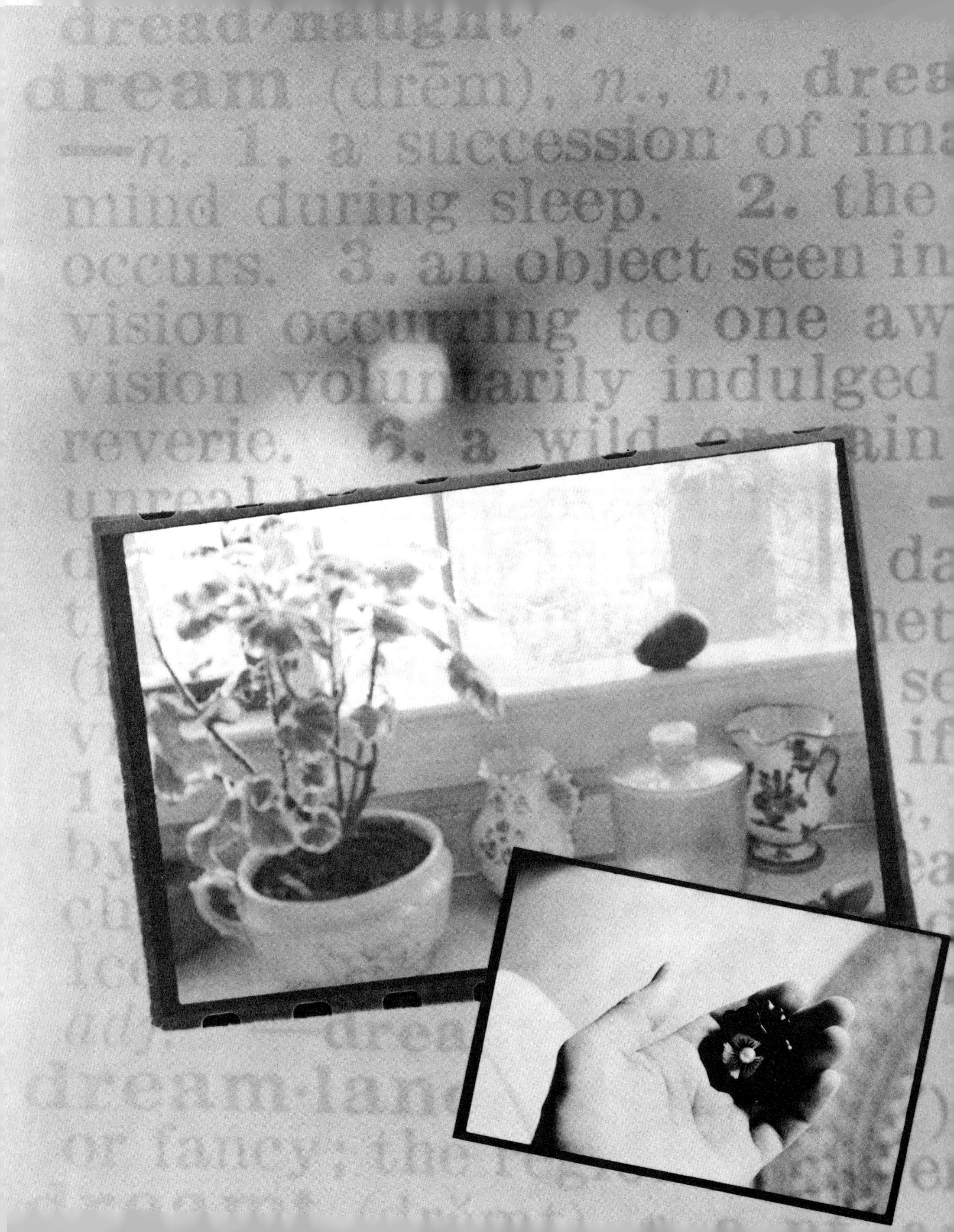
dream (drēm), n., v., drea
—n. 1. a succession of ima
mind during sleep. 2. the
occurs. 3. an object seen in
vision occurring to one aw
vision voluntarily indulged
reverie. a wild
dream·lan
or fancy; the

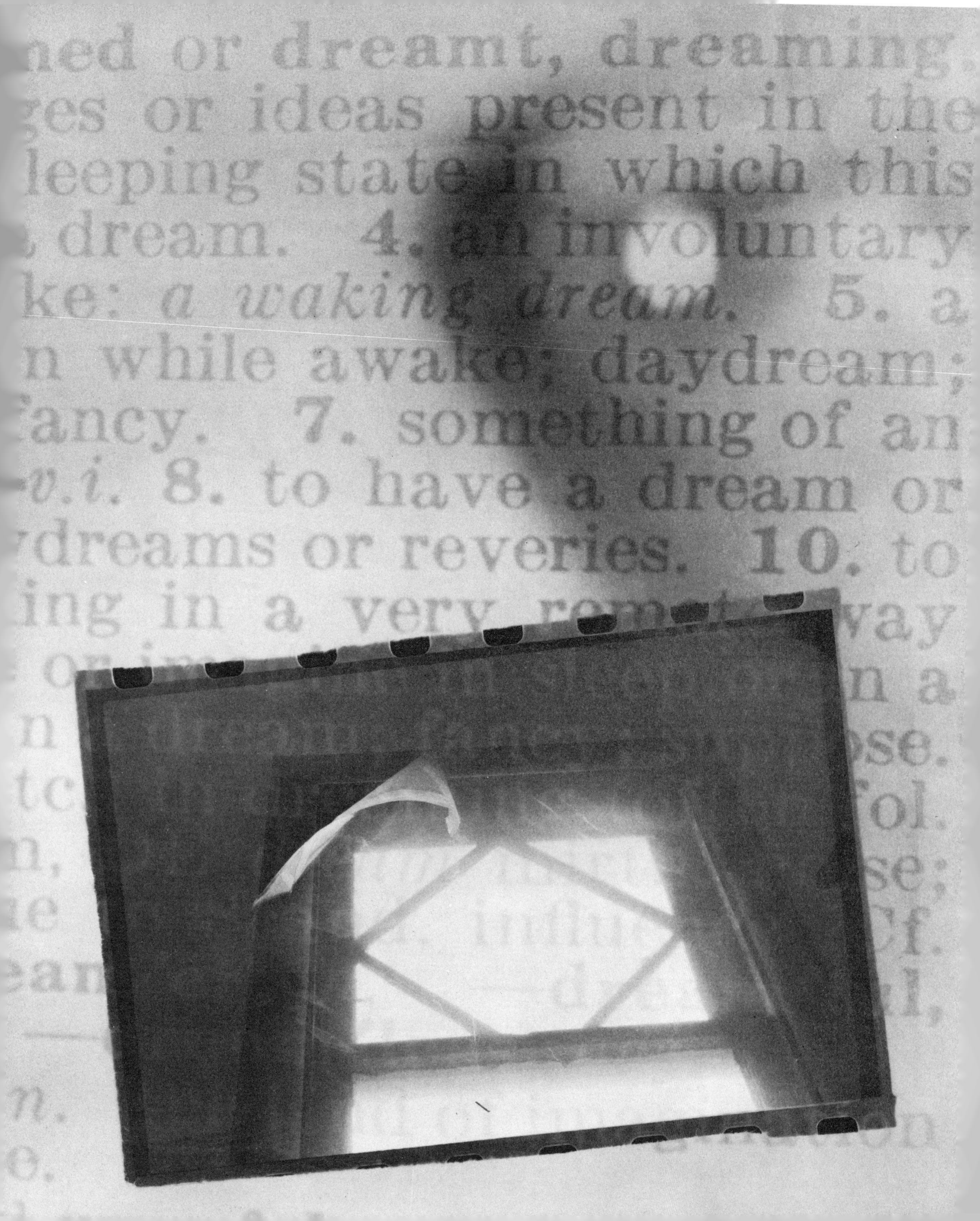
ned or dreamt, dreaming
ges or ideas present in the
leeping state in which this
dream. 4. an involuntary
ke: a waking dream. 5. a
n while awake; daydream;
ancy. 7. something of an
v.i. 8. to have a dream or
dreams or reveries. 10. to
ing in a very remote way

...; unformulated; poignant; supernatural; recurrent; indefinable; unfathomable; overwhelming; inspiring.

verbs
attend with—; awaken—; cause—; cure of—; diagnose—; disguise—; dwell in—; hide in—; indulge—; nourish—; obsess with—; oppress by—; overcome—; produce—; provoke—; put away—; regard with—; relinquish—; ripen into—; shake with—; wrap in—; —causes; —dogs; —inspires; —overcomes.
(See fright, horror, terror, awe.)

DREAD (♥)

adverbs
...; vaguely; habitually; superstitiously; ignorantly; apprehensively; unreasonably; secretly; speechlessly; shrinkingly; inexplicably; hauntingly; unimaginably; inexpressibly; morbidly; somberly; irrationally; starkly; mutually; constantly; unnaturally; foolishly; oppressively; vaguely; nervously; piously; poignantly; supernaturally; recurrently; indefinably; unfathomably; overwhelmingly.
(See fear, anticipate.)

DREADFUL

adverbs
unutterably; unspeakably; horridly; abominably; tragically; gloomily; incredibly; indescribably; absolutely; starkly; uncommonly; amazingly; astonishingly; cruelly; shockingly; startlingly; perniciously; damnably; disastrously; ruinously ...

...ic; drowsy; embodied; empty; enthralled; external; evil; exacerbated; exquisite; extraordinary; extravagant; exuberant; fabulous; faded; fairy tale; false; fanatical; fanciful; fancy; fantastic; favorite; fearful; feverish; fitful; flashing; flattering; fleeting; floating; fond; foolish; fragile; friendly; frightful; futile; ghastly; girlish; glorious; gloomy; golden; gorgeous; grandiose; grotesque; half-forgotten; half-remembered; hashish; hateful; haunting; hazy; hideous; horrible; horrid; horrifying; hovering; idle; idyllic; illusory; immortal; impossible; impressive; incommunicable; industrial; ineffaceable; ingenuous; insistent; inspiring; interlunar; interminable; intransitive; invisible; iridescent; jeweled; jostling; journeying; jocund; languorous; lasting; lethargic; liquored; lifelong; liberal-minded; living; loftiest; lotus-eating; lowly; luxurious; mad; maddening; magical; magnificent; melancholy; materialized; millennial; misty; mournful; mooning; morbid; nightly; nightmare; obliging; particular; pensive; perfectible; perishing; odorous; oppressive; ominous; painful; perpetual; persistent; picturesque; pipe; poetic; pompous; poor; preposterous; prophetic; quarrelsome; protracted; pure; quaint; quaking; qualm-filled; quarrelsome; quavering; queenly; quenchable; quick; quieting; querimonious; querulous; questionable; quirky; quizzical; ... restless; resurr...

produce—; realize—; rule—; shake off—; shatter—; sink into—; slumber in—; spin—; suffer in—; transform—; understand—; wander in—; —betokens; —crumbles; —disturbs; —flees; —flowers; —foretells; —haunts; —overpowers; —overshadows; —presages; —prophesies; —puzzles; —reveals; —signifies; —startles; —terrifies; —torments; —troubles; —warns.
(See illusion, reverie, fancy, fantasy, hallucination, vision.)

DREAM (♥)

adverbs
unchastely; delectably; romantically; splendidly; confusedly; fondly; contentedly; ambitiously; amusingly; astonishingly; blissfully; dazzlingly; deliciously; deliriously; disconnectedly; drowsily; distressingly; dreadfully; ecstatically; emptily; evilly; exquisitely; extravagantly; exuberantly; fabulously; fanatically; fancifully; fleetingly; gloomily; gorgeously; grotesquely; horribly; inspiringly; interminably; maddeningly; magnificently; oppressively; pensively; perpetually; persistently; picturesquely; poetically; prophetically; ridiculously; romantically; senselessly; sensually; significantly; vividly; waveringly; zestfully; deliriously.
(S... ...ine.)

DREAMER

... preposterous; imagin... ...mpractical; hair-split... ...; soppy; deep; bliss... ...; superstitious; un...

DREAMY

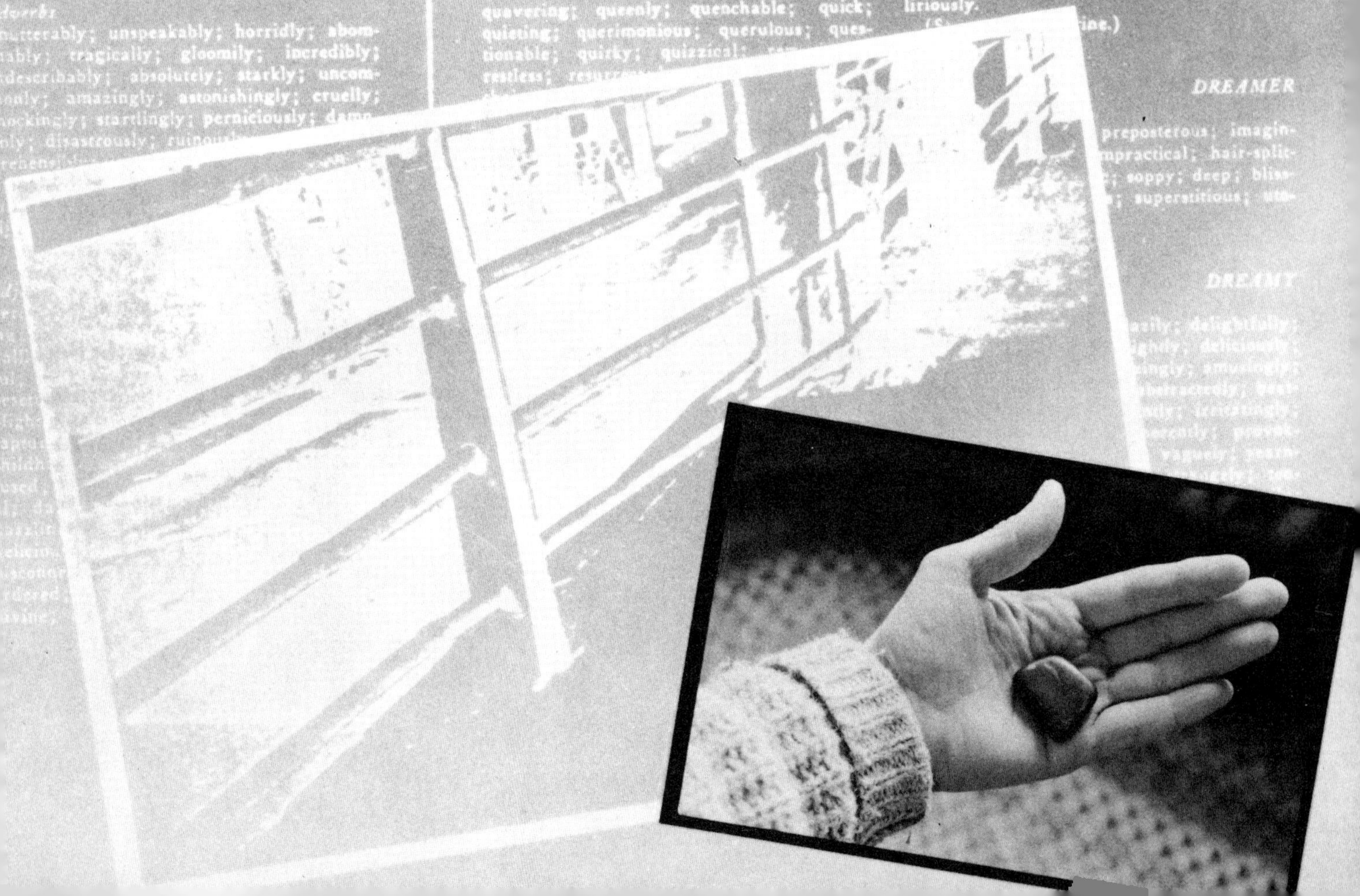

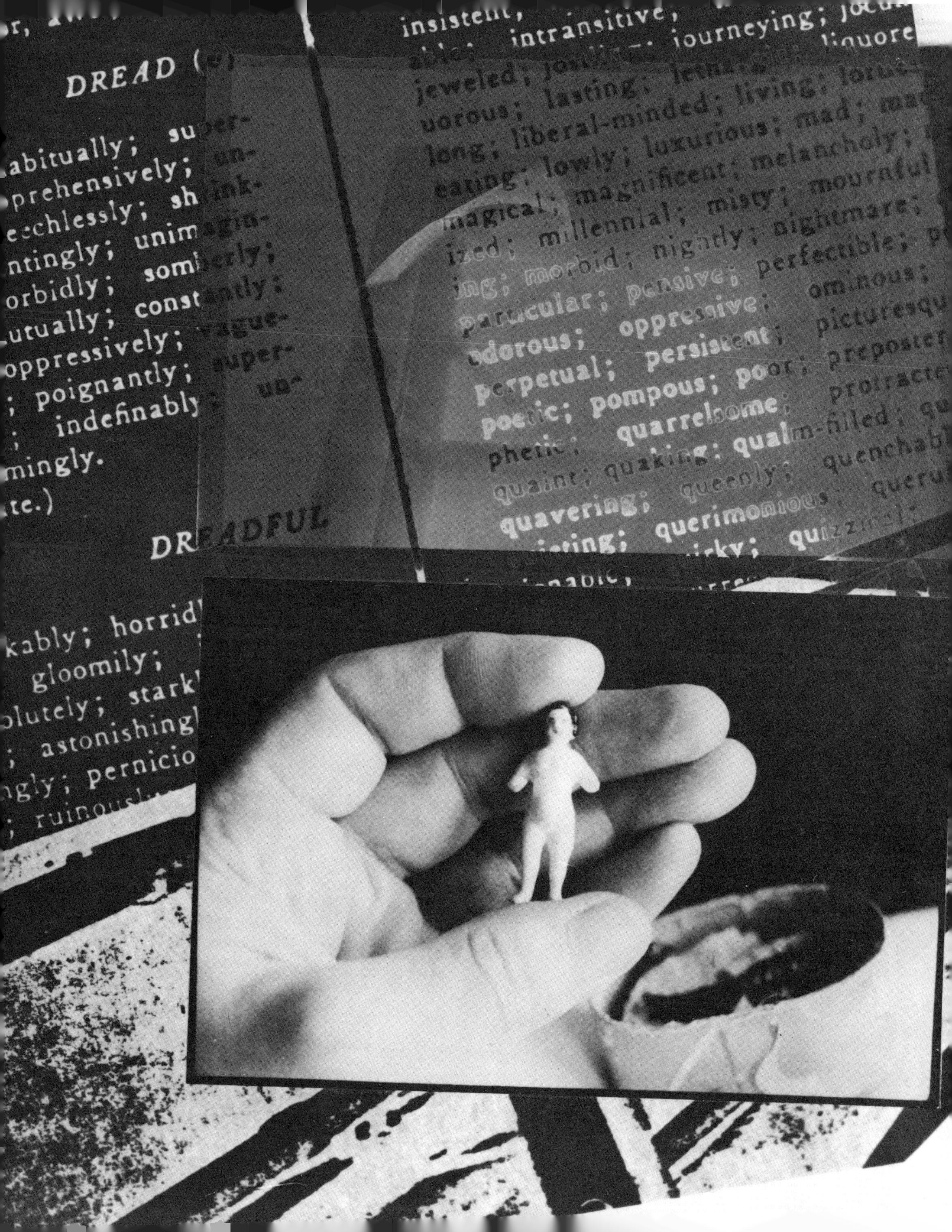
DREAD
DREADFUL
insistent; intransitive; journeying;
jeweled; lasting;
long; liberal-minded; living;
lowly; luxurious; mad;
magnificent; melancholy;
magical; millennial; misty; mournful
nightly; nightmare;
morbid; perfectible;
particular; pensive; ominous;
odorous; oppressive; picturesque
perpetual; persistent; preposter
poetic; pompous; poor; protract
quarrelsome; qualm-filled;
quaint; quaking; quenchab
queenly;
quavering; querimonious
querimonious; quizzic
prehensively;
eechlessly;
ntingly; unimagin-
orbidly; somberly;
utually; constantly;
oppressively; vague-
poignantly; super-
indefinably; un-
mingly.
kably; horrid
gloomily;
olutely; stark
astonishing
ngly; pernicio
ruinous

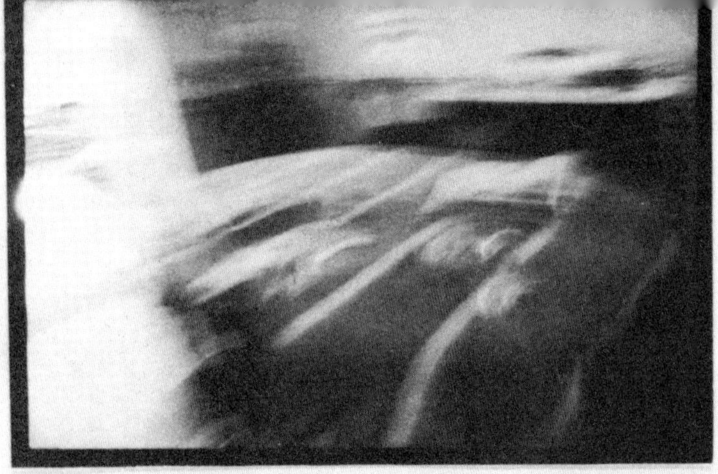
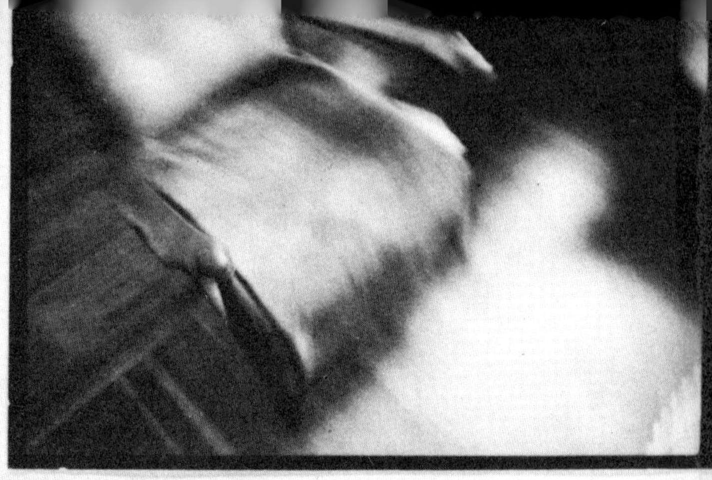
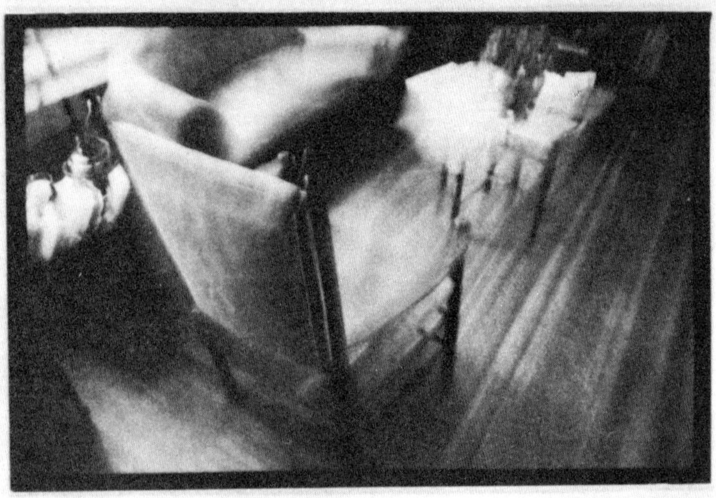
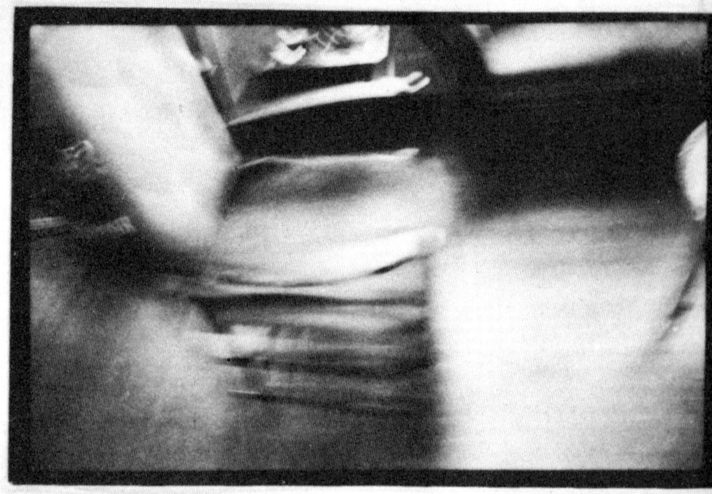
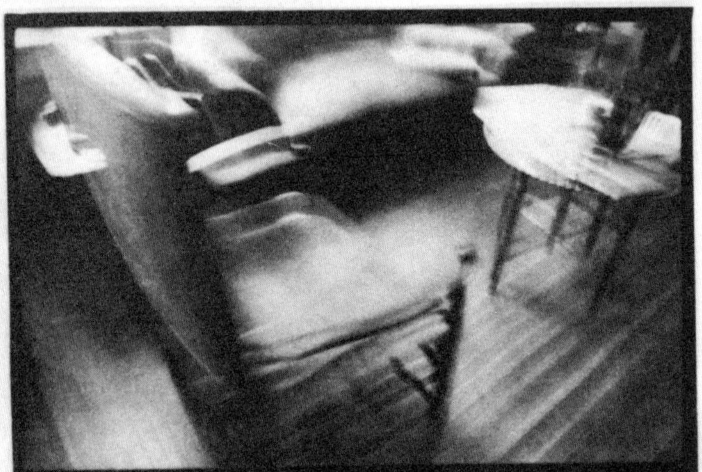
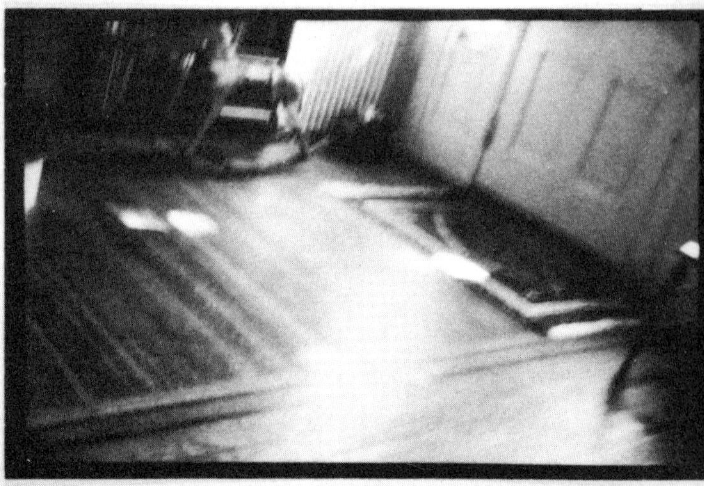
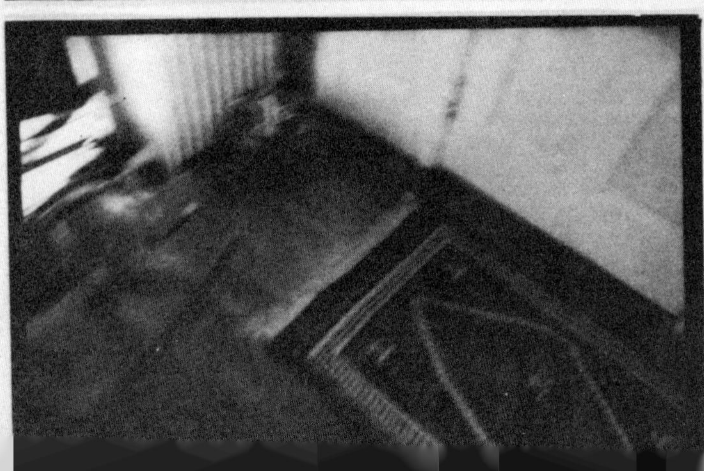
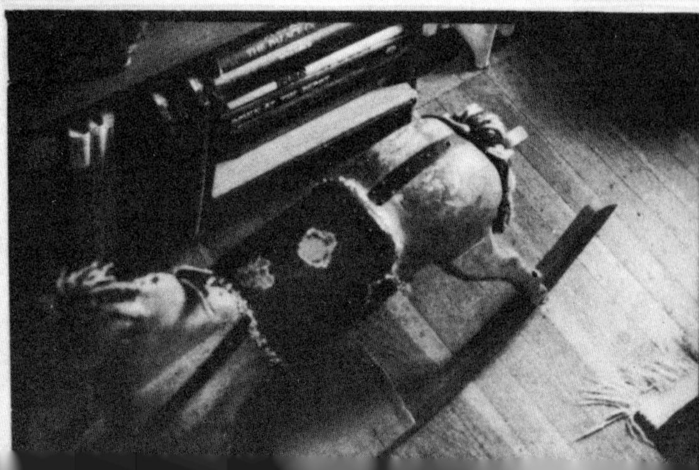

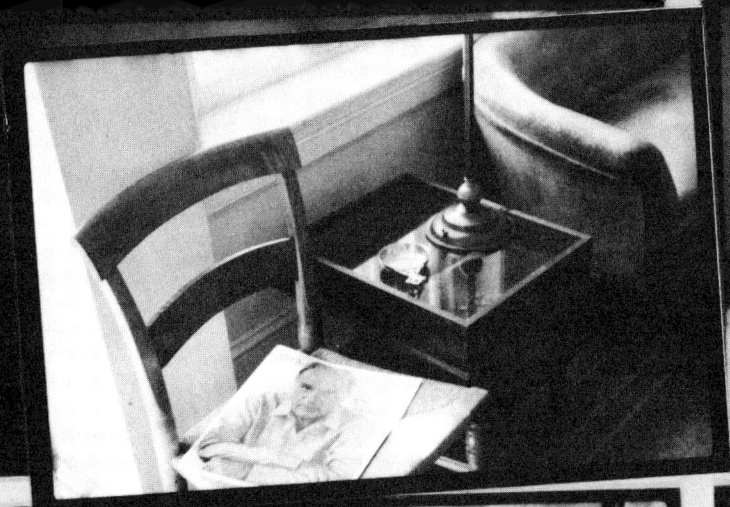

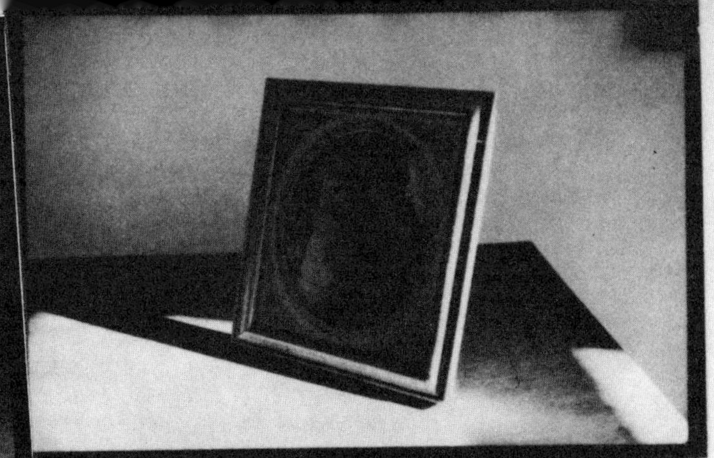

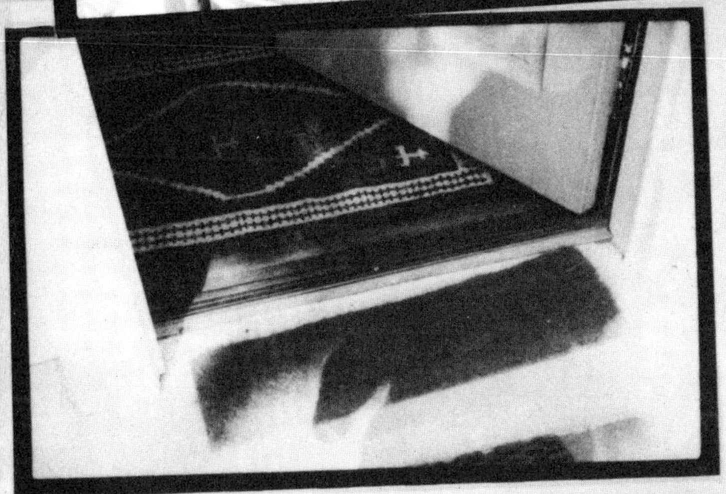

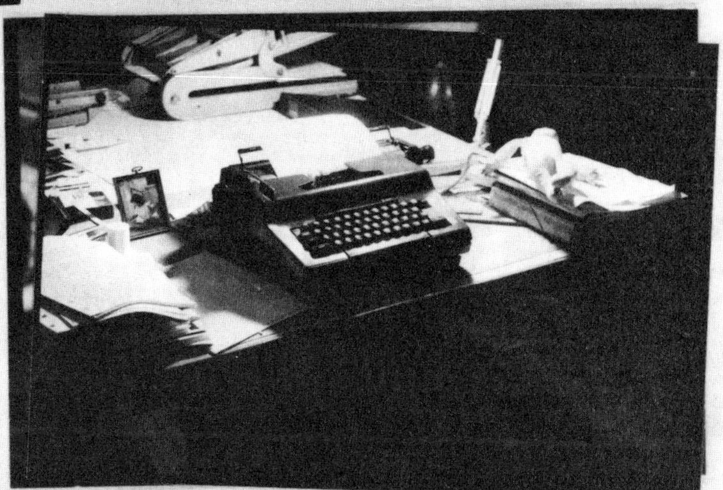

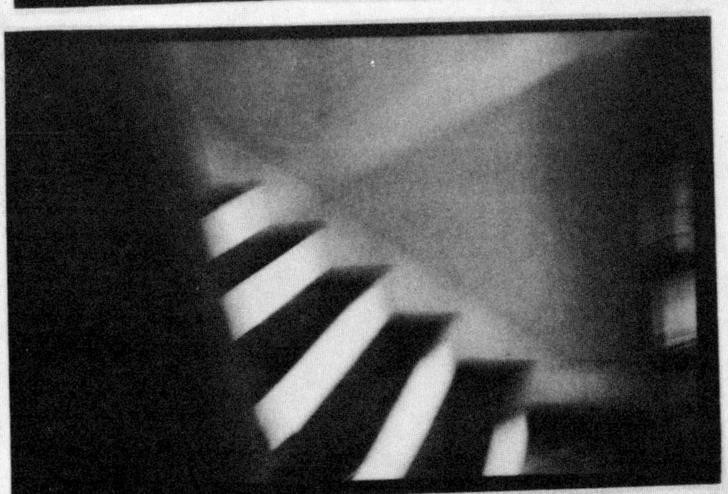

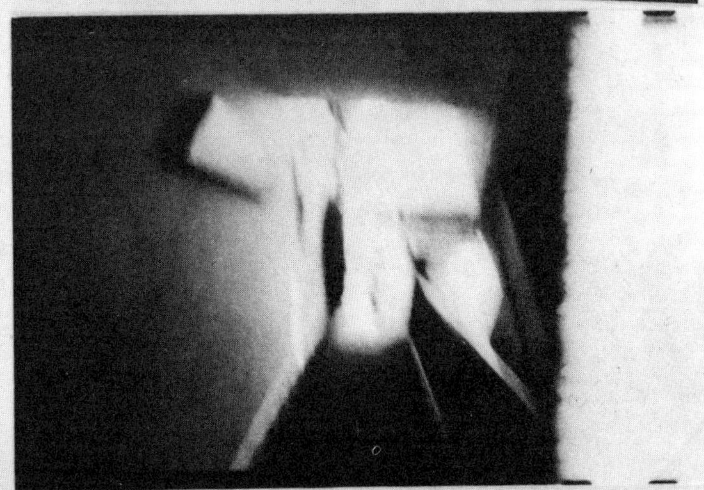

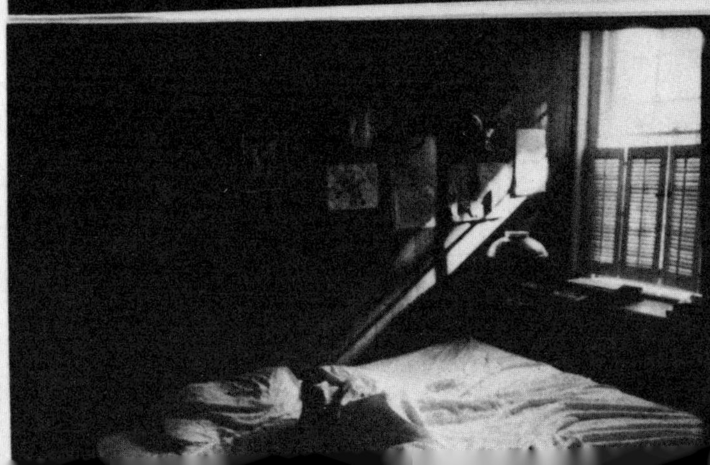

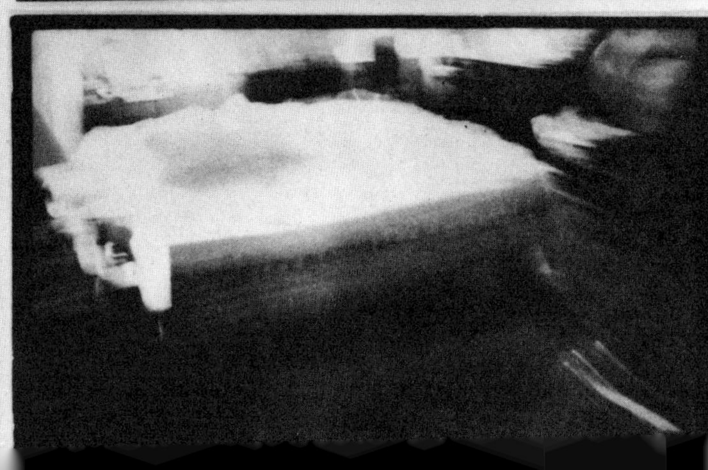

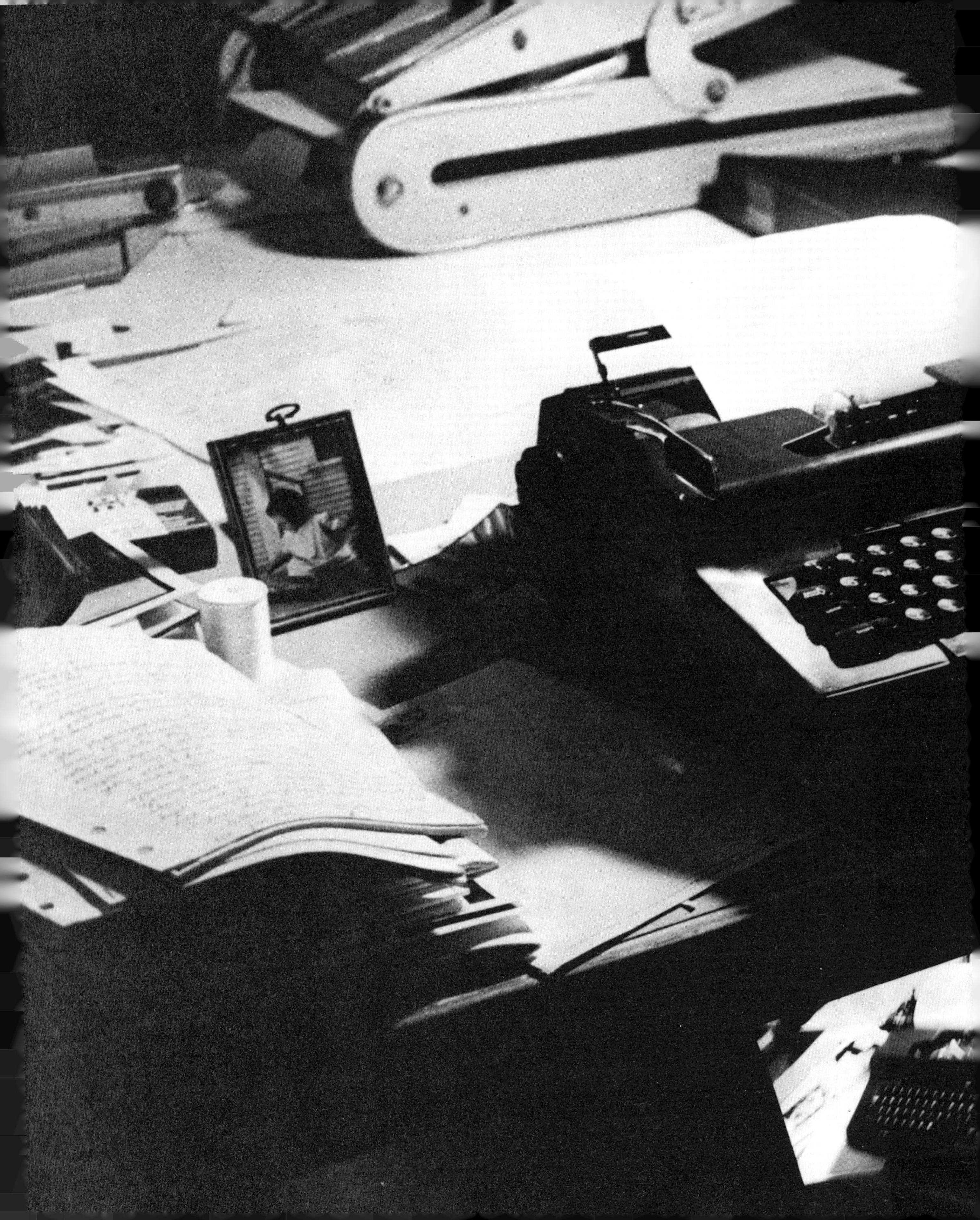

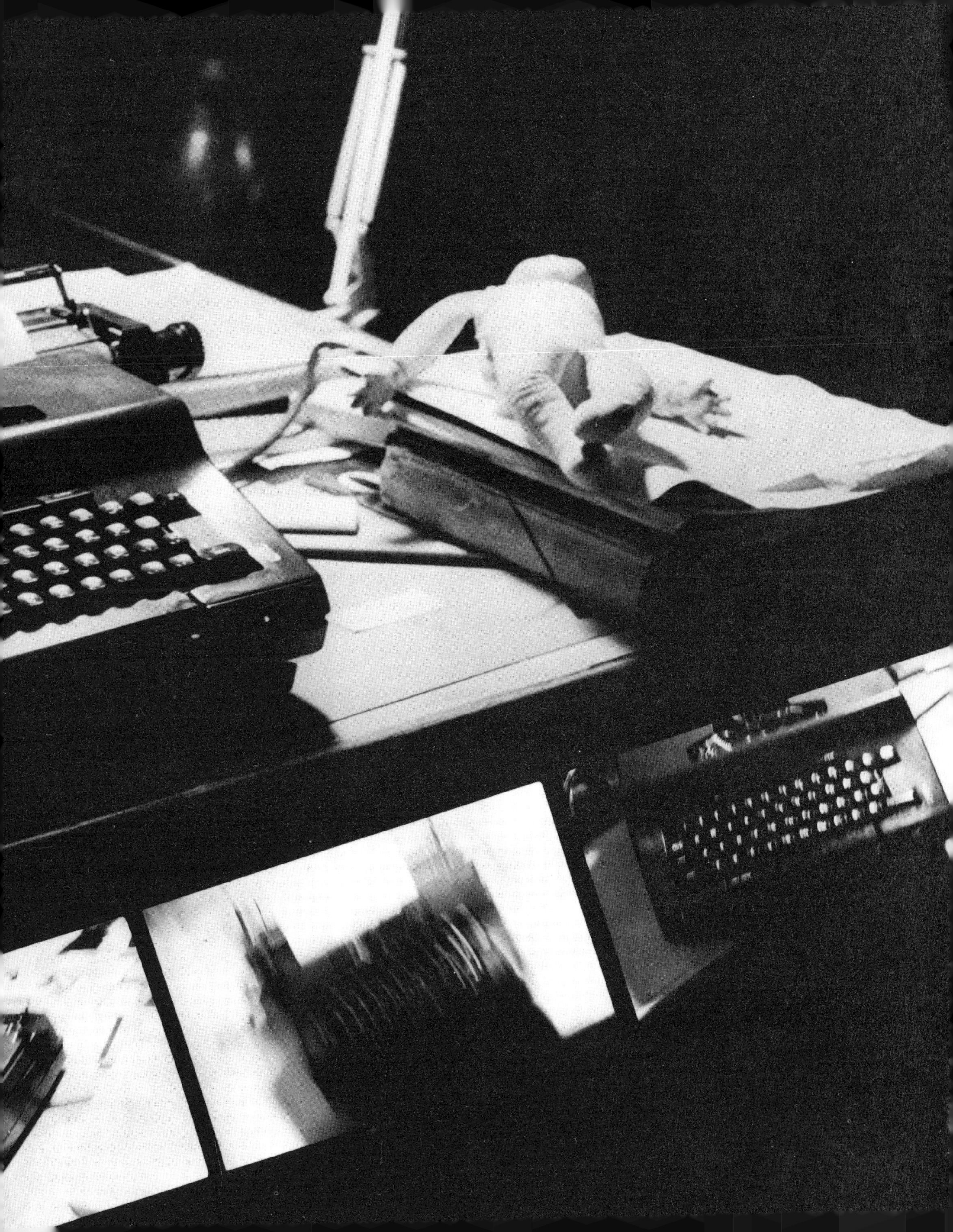

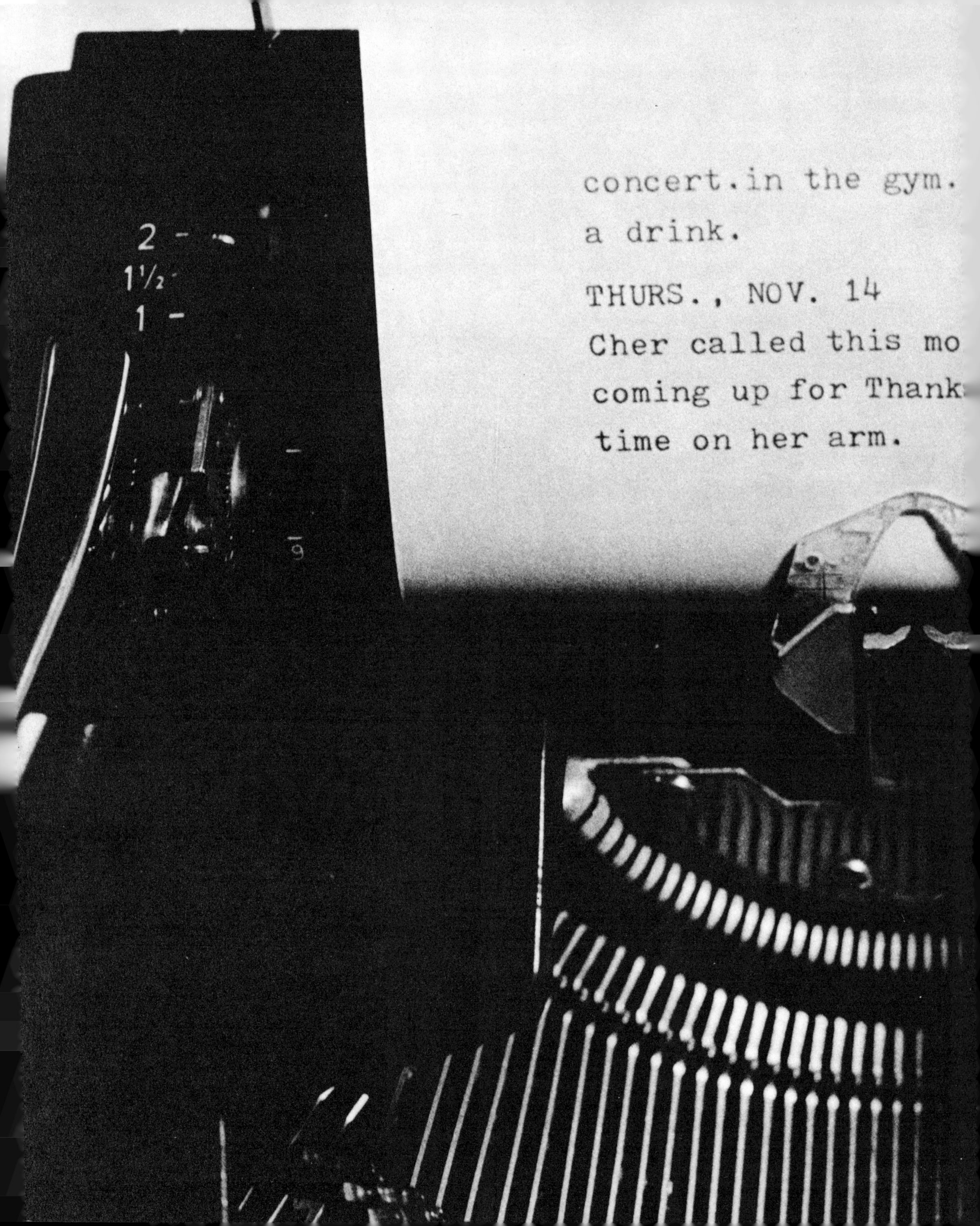
2 -
1½
1 -
concert.in the gym.
a drink.
THURS., NOV. 14
Cher called this mo
coming up for Thank
time on her arm.

Went to Lois and Duryea's afterward for

ng to tell me she and Melissa won't be
ving. The melanoma has reappeared, this

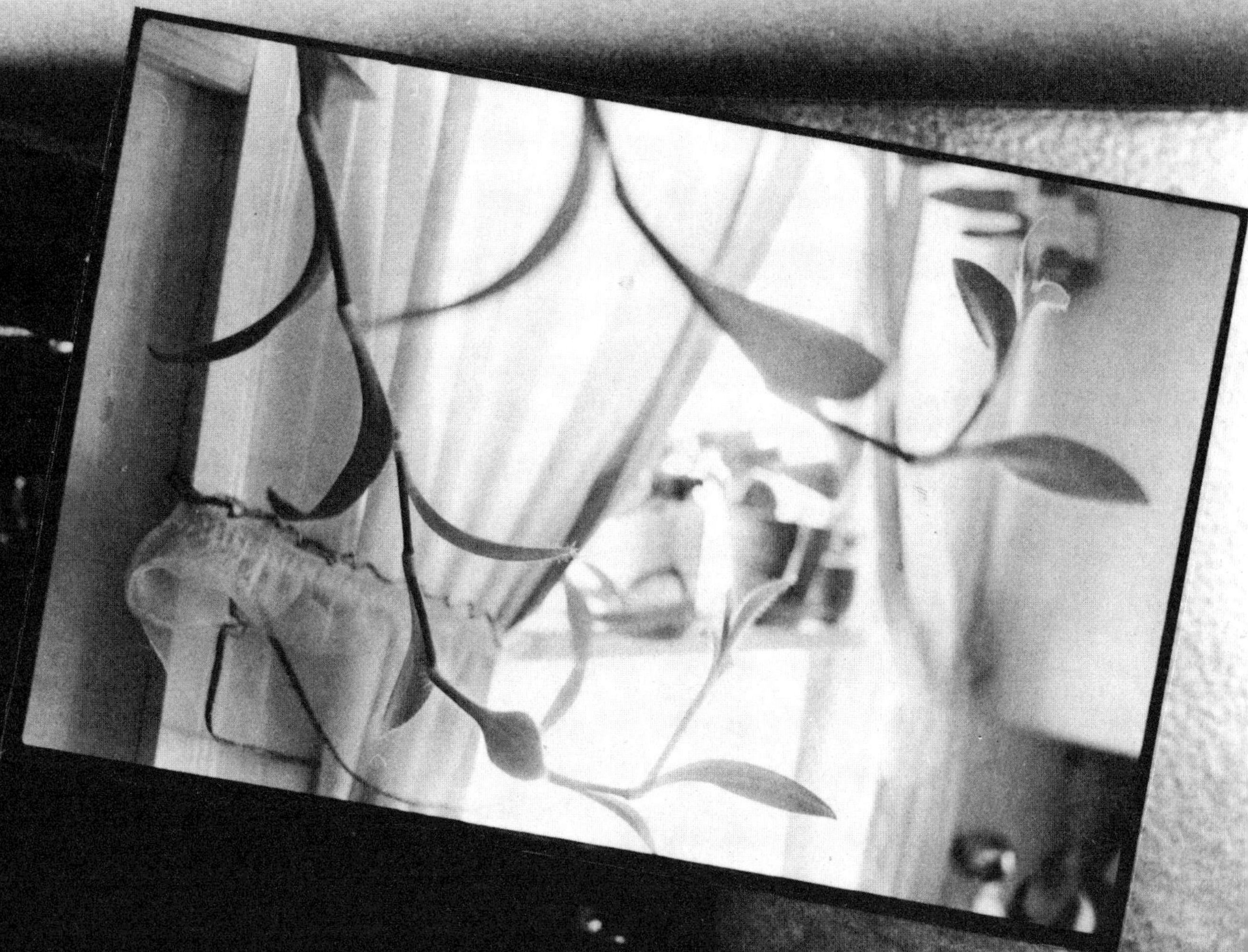

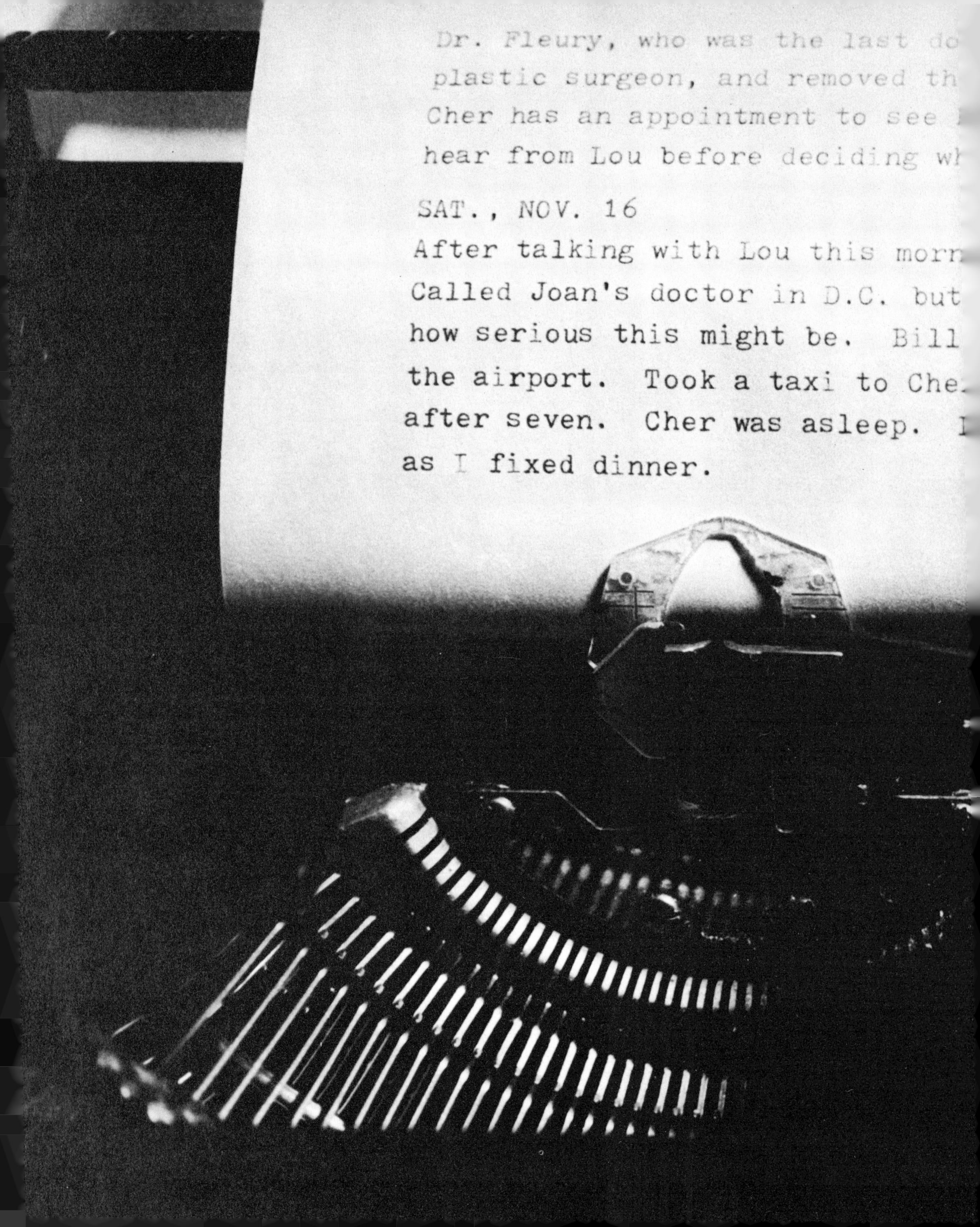
Dr. Fleury, who was the last do
plastic surgeon, and removed th
Cher has an appointment to see
hear from Lou before deciding wh
SAT., NOV. 16
After talking with Lou this morn
Called Joan's doctor in D.C. but
how serious this might be. Bill
the airport. Took a taxi to Che
after seven. Cher was asleep.
as I fixed dinner.

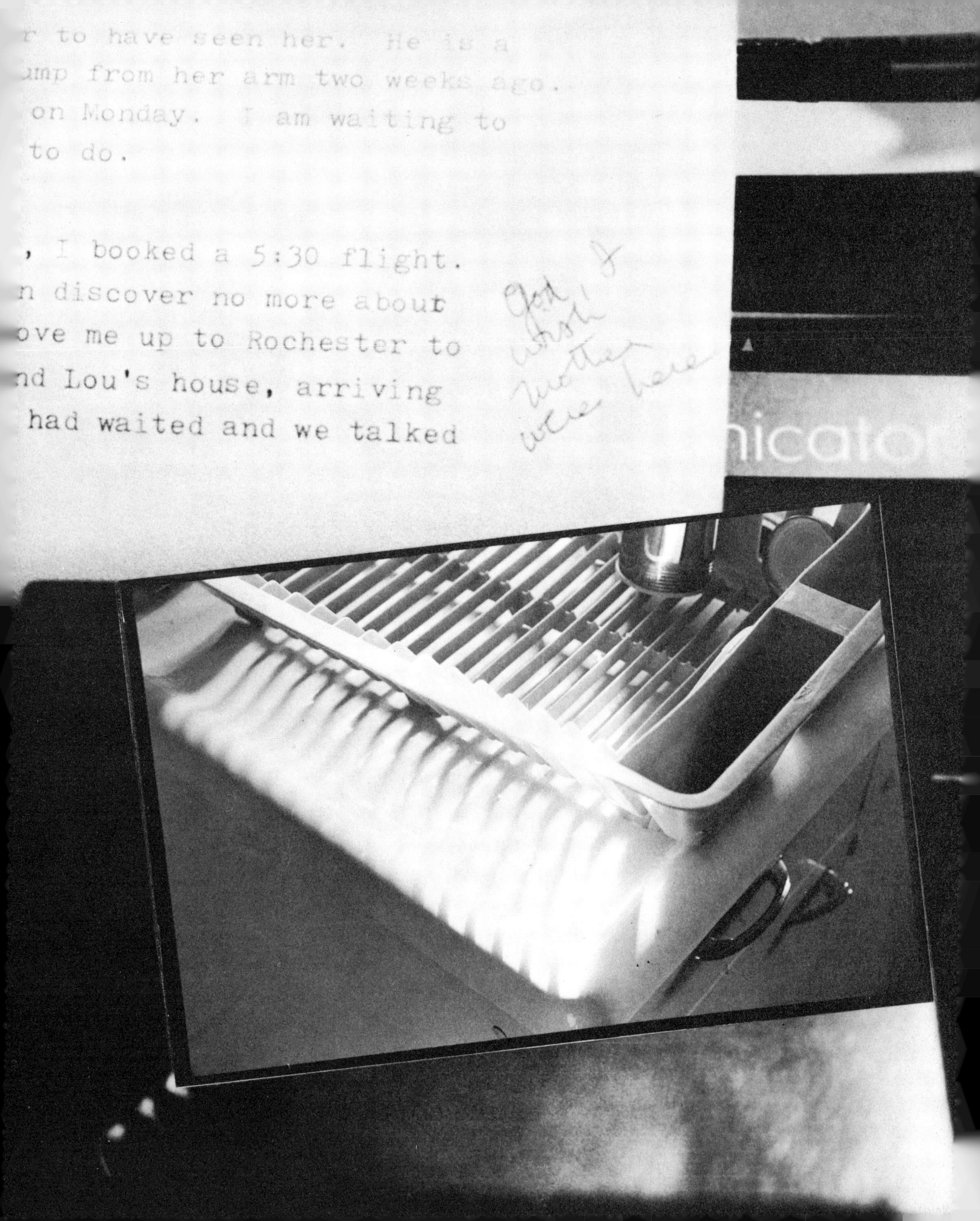
r to have seen her. He is a
ump from her arm two weeks ago.
on Monday. I am waiting to
to do.
, I booked a 5:30 flight.
n discover no more about
ove me up to Rochester to
nd Lou's house, arriving
had waited and we talked
nicato

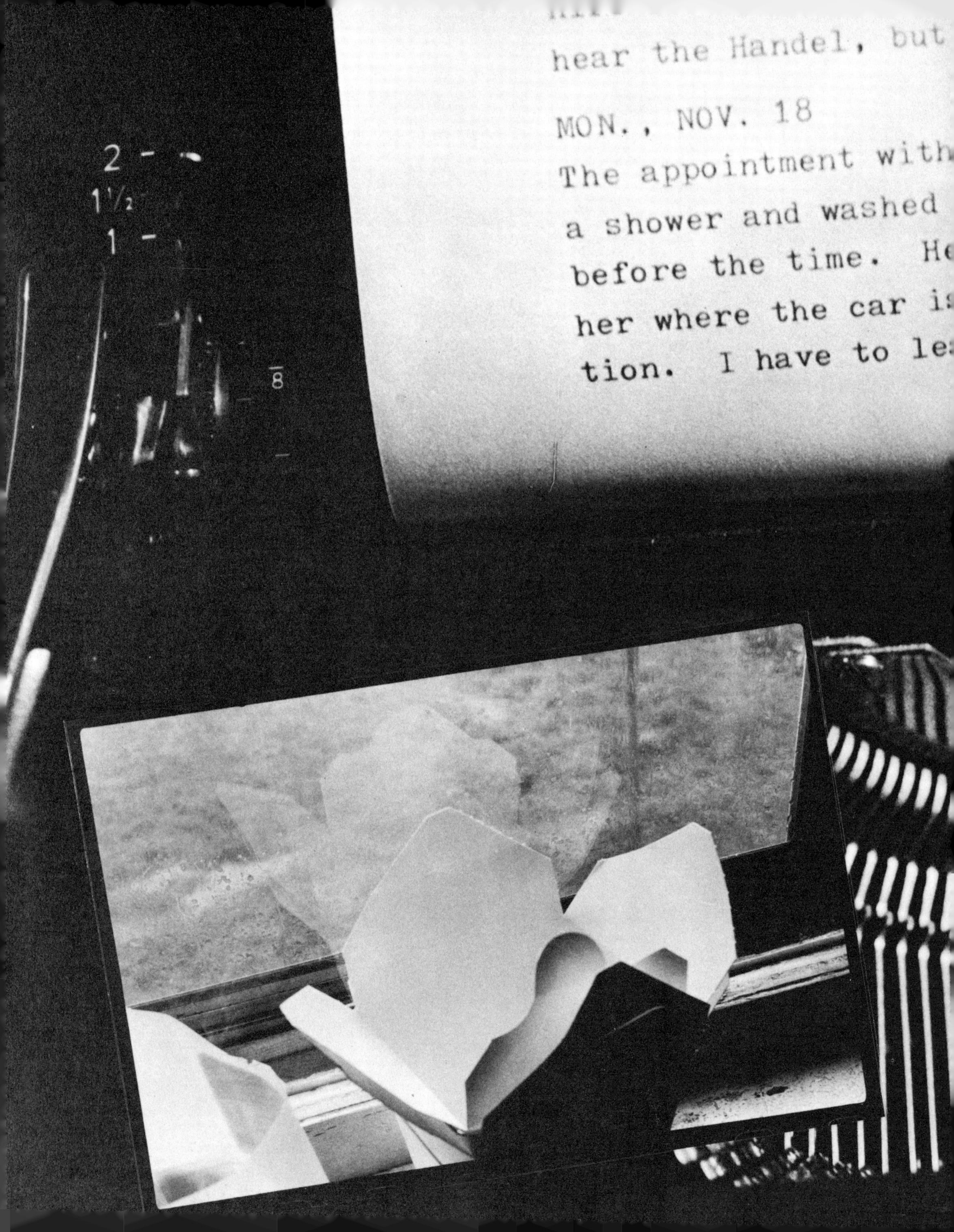
hear the Handel, but
MON., NOV. 18
The appointment with
a shower and washed
before the time.
her where the car
tion. I have to

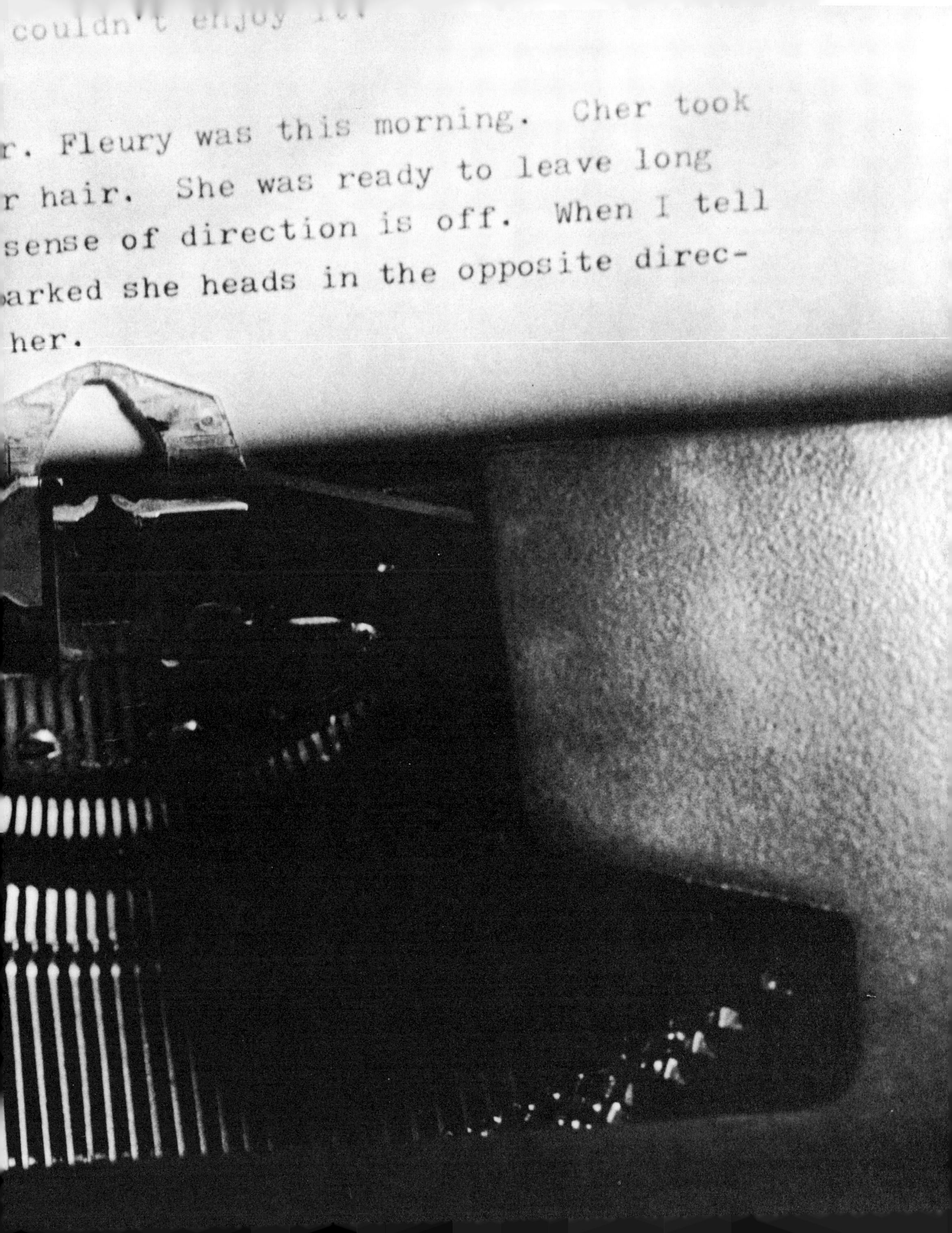
couldn't enjoy
r. Fleury was this morning. Cher took
r hair. She was ready to leave long
sense of direction is off. When I tell
arked she heads in the opposite direc-
her.

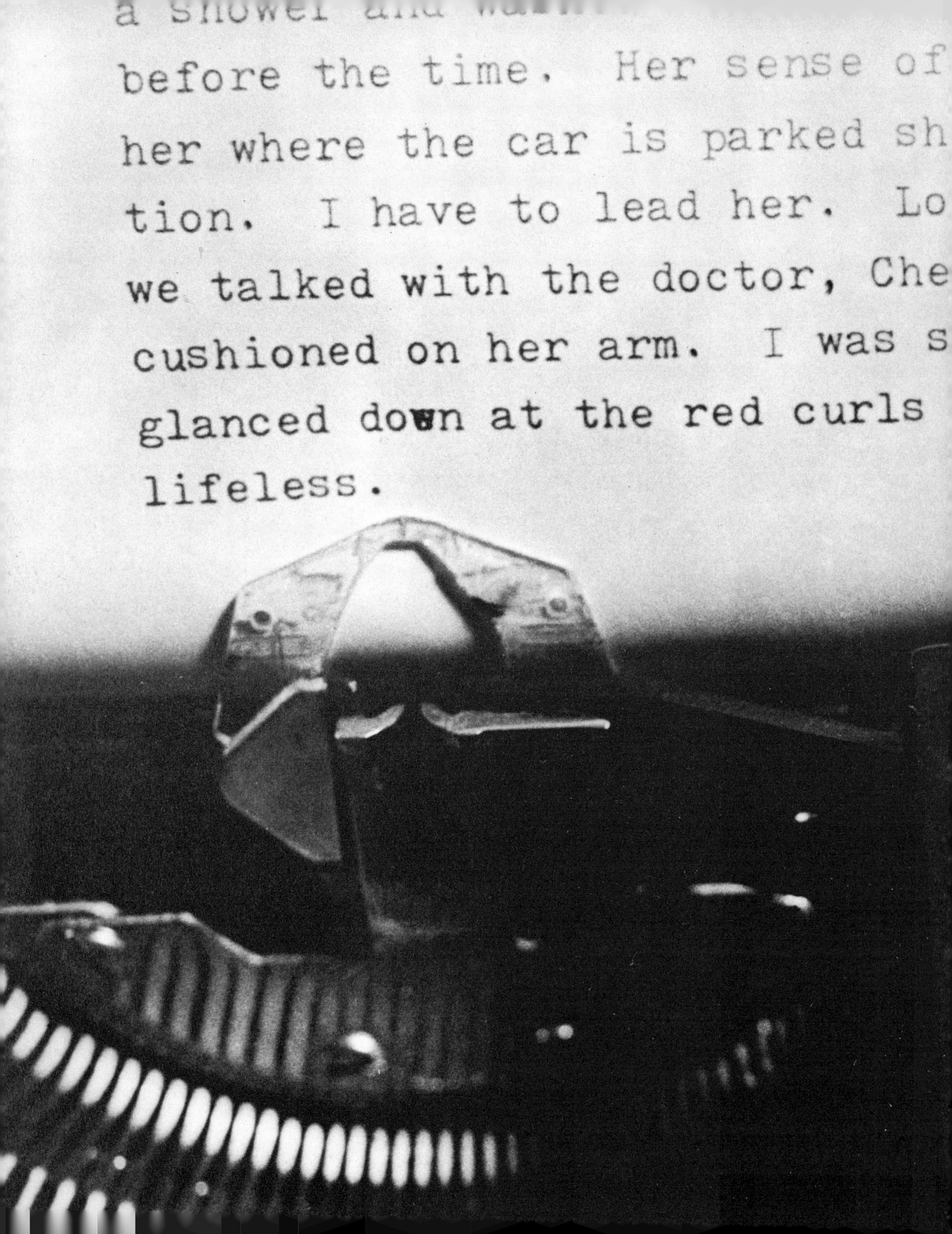
before the time. Her sense of
her where the car is parked sh
tion. I have to lead her. Lo
we talked with the doctor, Che
cushioned on her arm. I was s
glanced down at the red curls
lifeless.

irection is off. When I tell
heads in the opposite direc-
met us at the office. While
sat with her head down,
cting just behind her and
e had just washed. They are

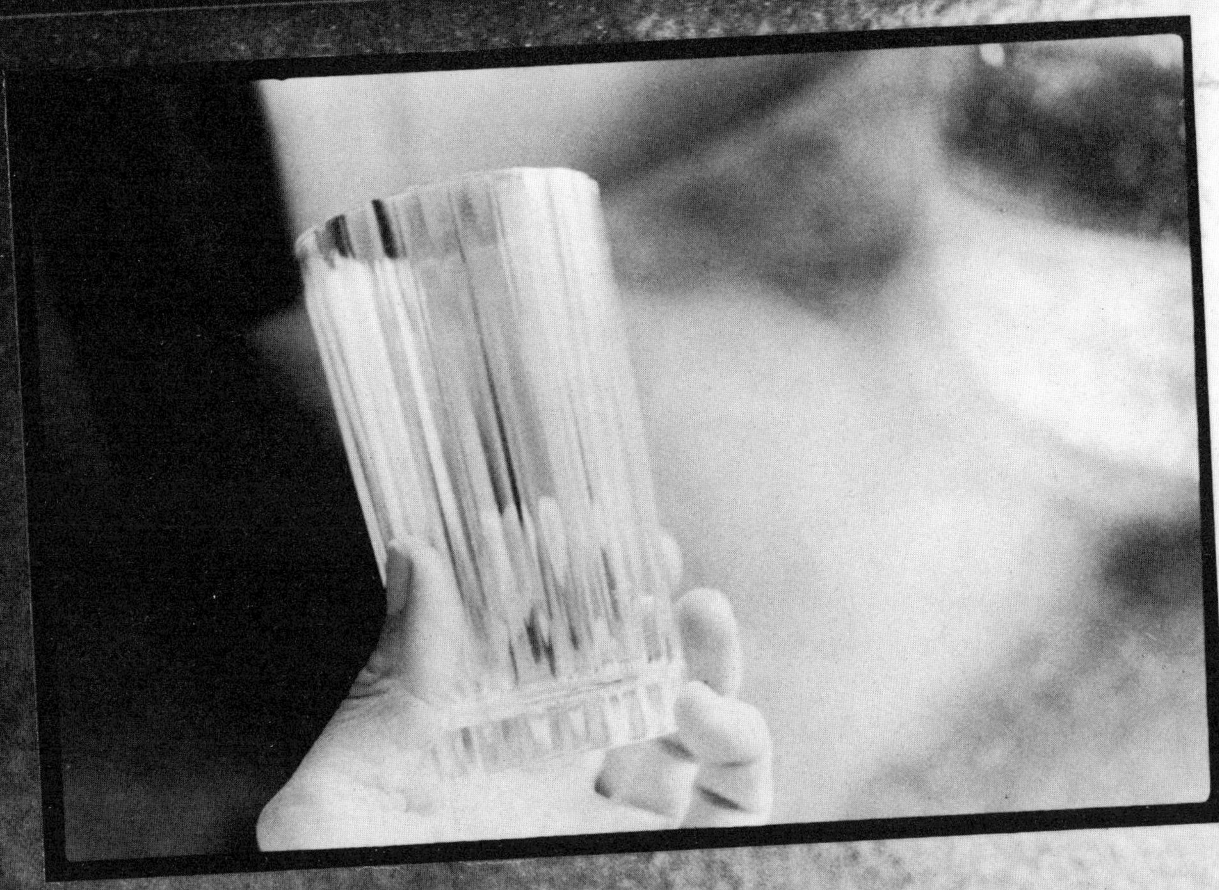

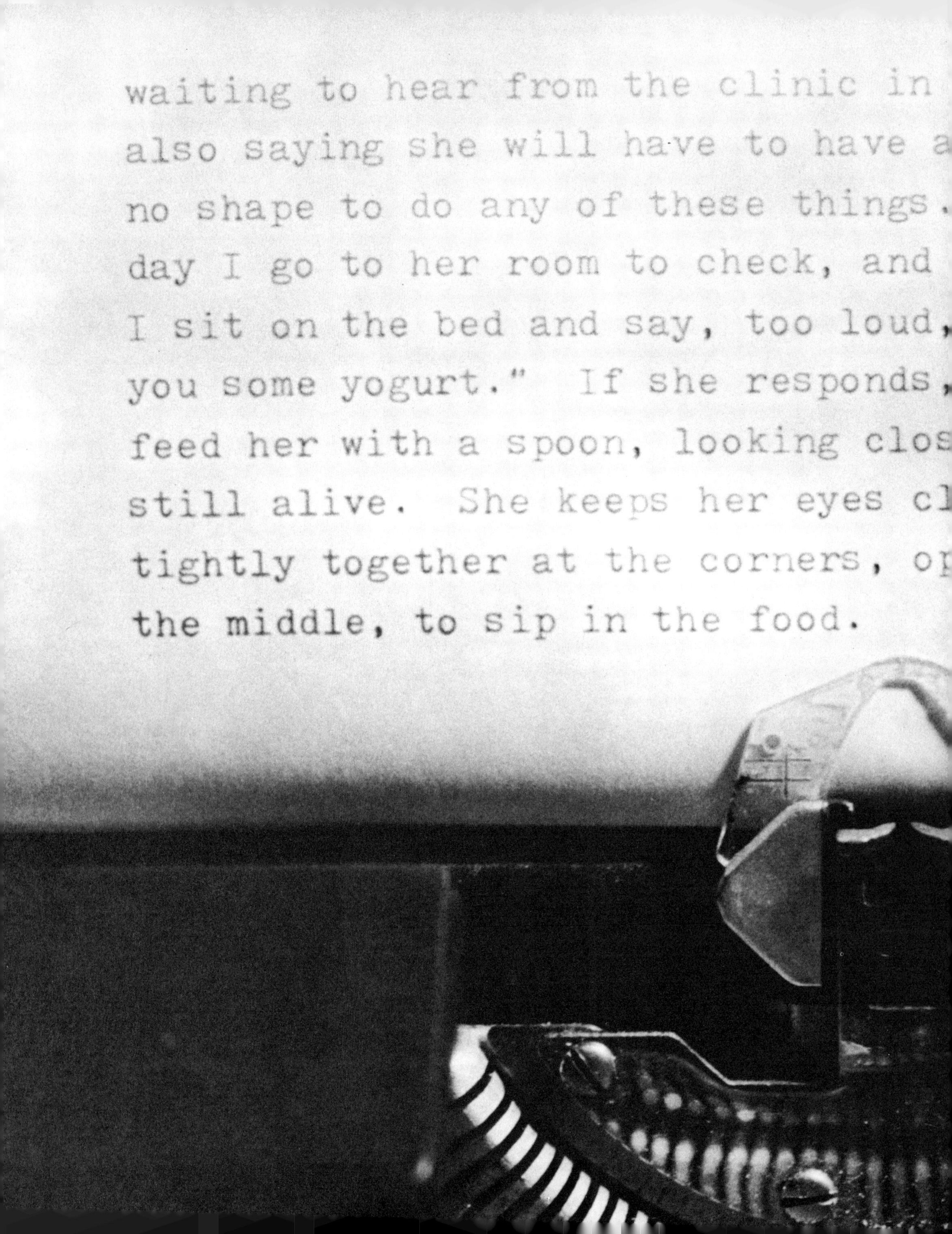

waiting to hear from the clinic in
also saying she will have to have a
no shape to do any of these things.
day I go to her room to check, and
I sit on the bed and say, too loud,
you some yogurt." If she responds,
feed her with a spoon, looking clos
still alive. She keeps her eyes cl
tightly together at the corners, op
the middle, to sip in the food.

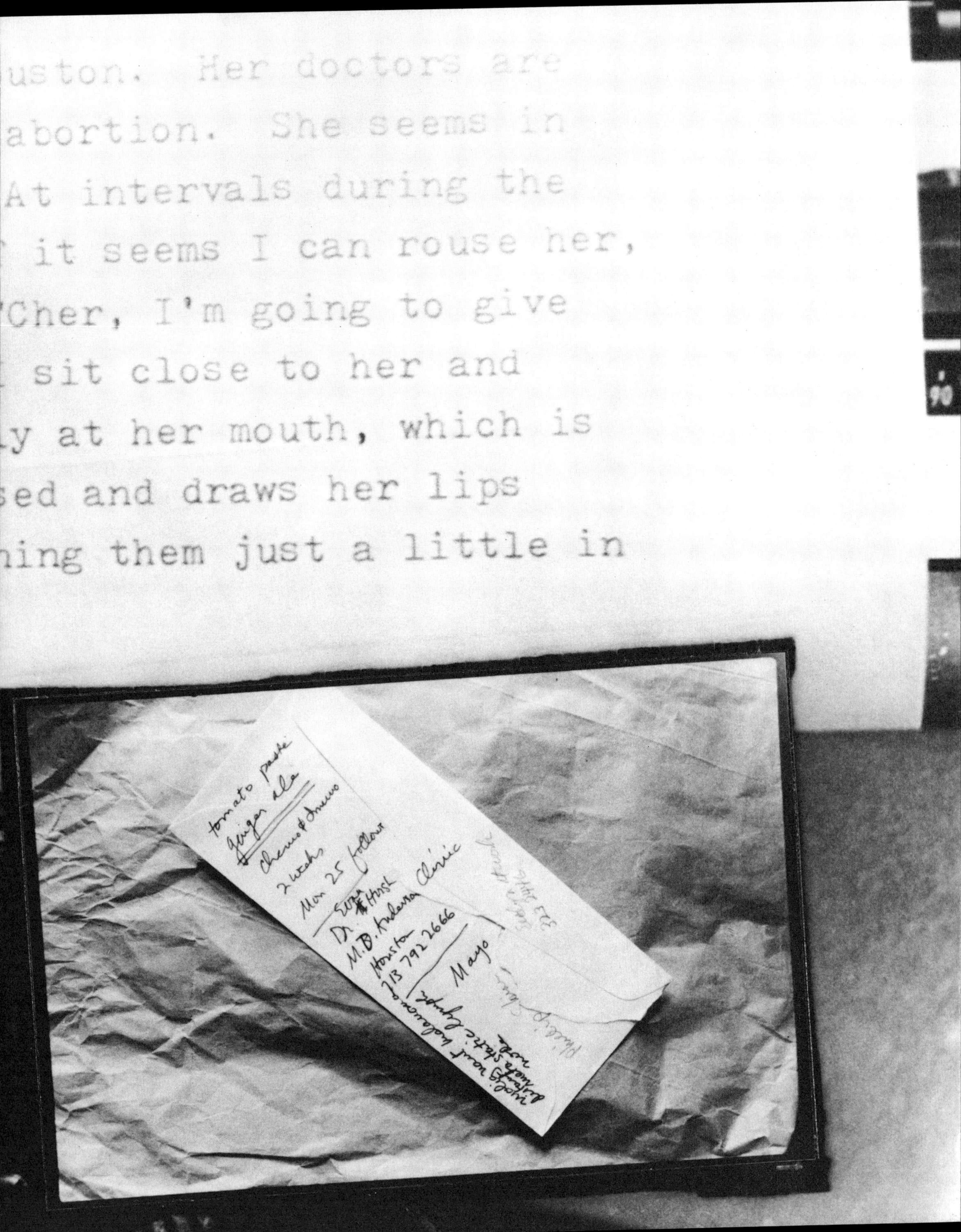
uston. Her doctors are
abortion. She seems in
At intervals during the
it seems I can rouse her,
Cher, I'm going to give
sit close to her and
y at her mouth, which is
sed and draws her lips
ning them just a little in
tomato paste
Ginger ale
Mon 25 follow
M.D. Anderson Clinic
Houston
713 792 2666
Mayo

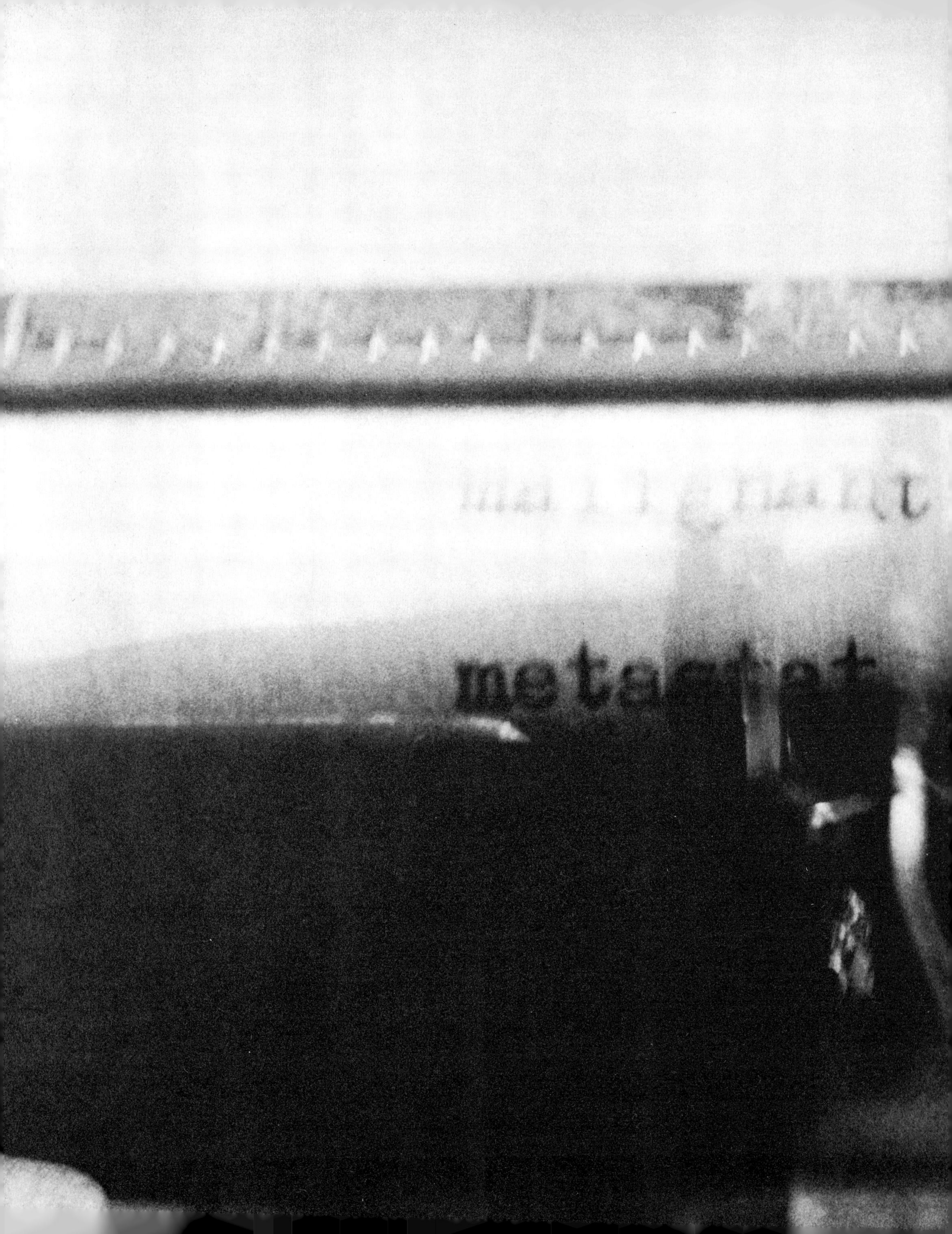

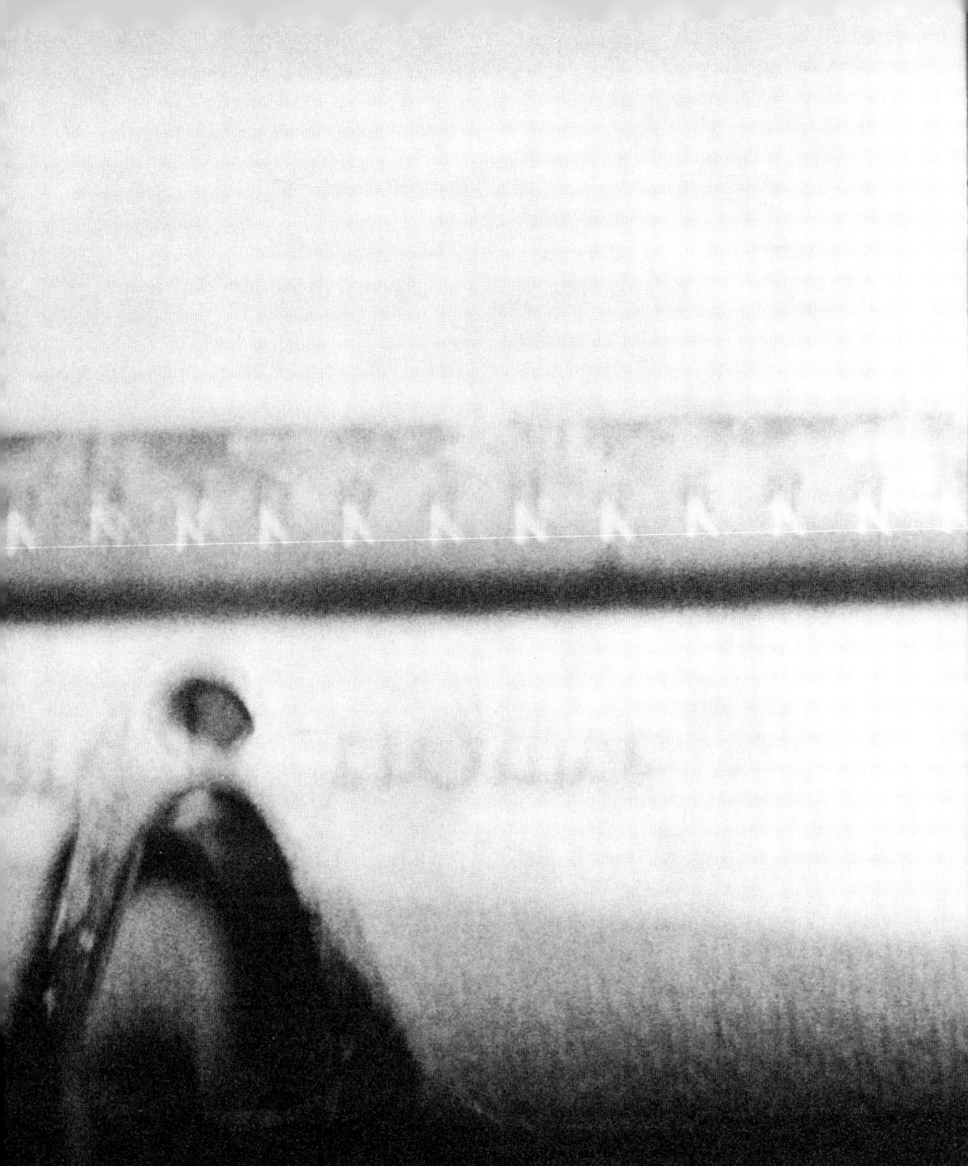

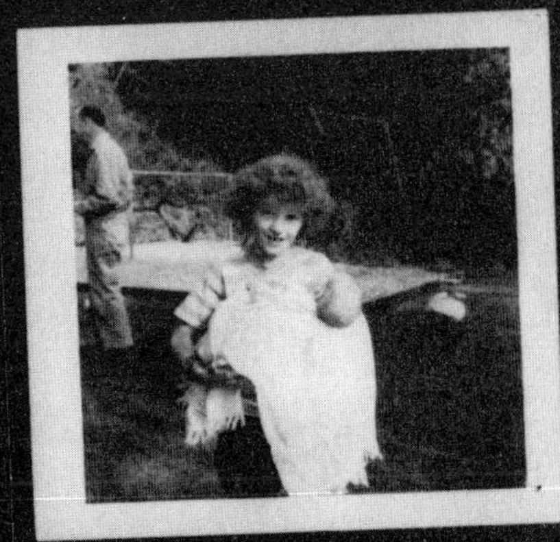

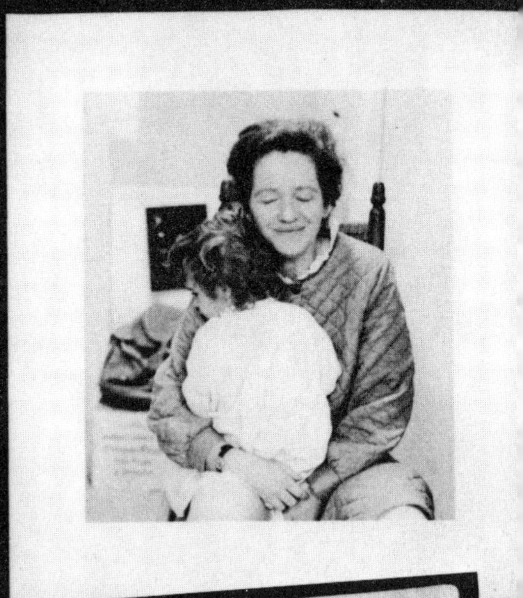

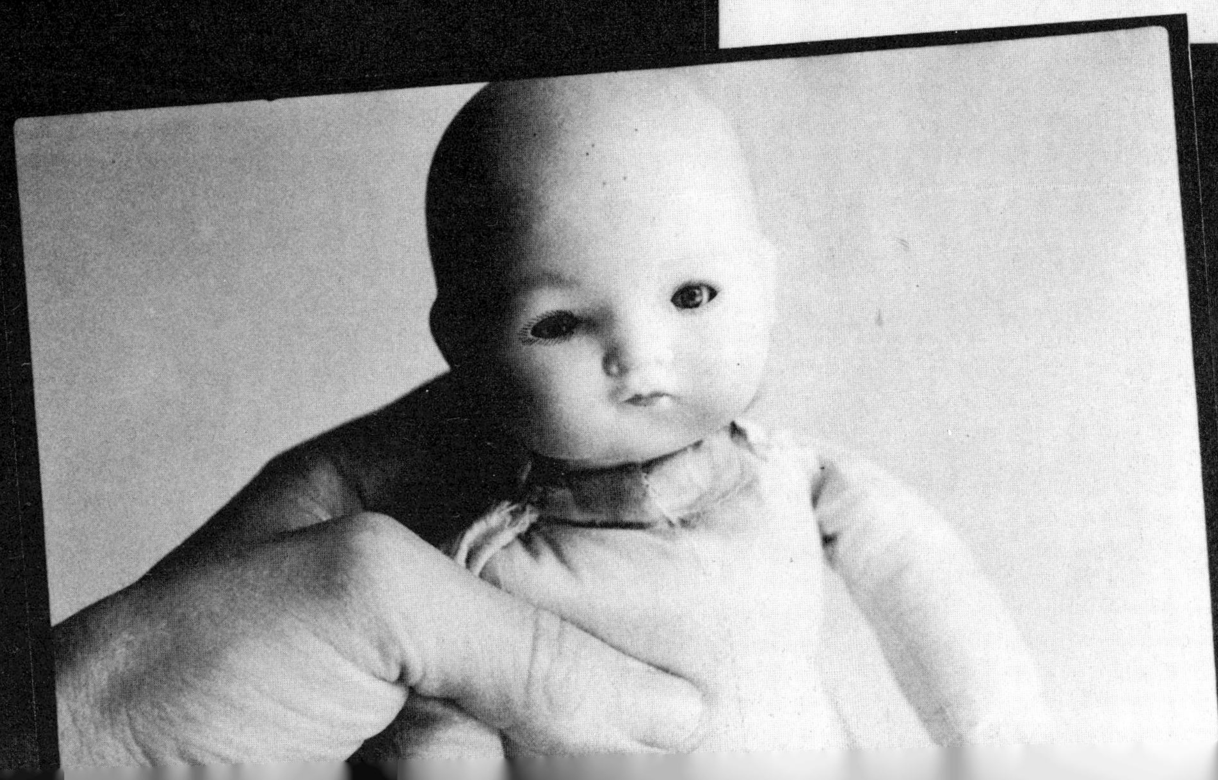

you some yogu

her with a spoon, looking closely at her mo

alive. She keeps hwr eyes closed and draws

together at the corners, opening them just

middle, to sip in the food. She says her h

give her asperin. All my efforts seem so

nor I feel we are able to reach her.

TUES., NOV. 19

Kathy drove us to Dr. Thomas office. Cher

drunk anything for twelve hours because th

lab work done. Her throat was parched, an

lay on the back seat of the VW bug, scrunc

table. We got lost in the one-way streets

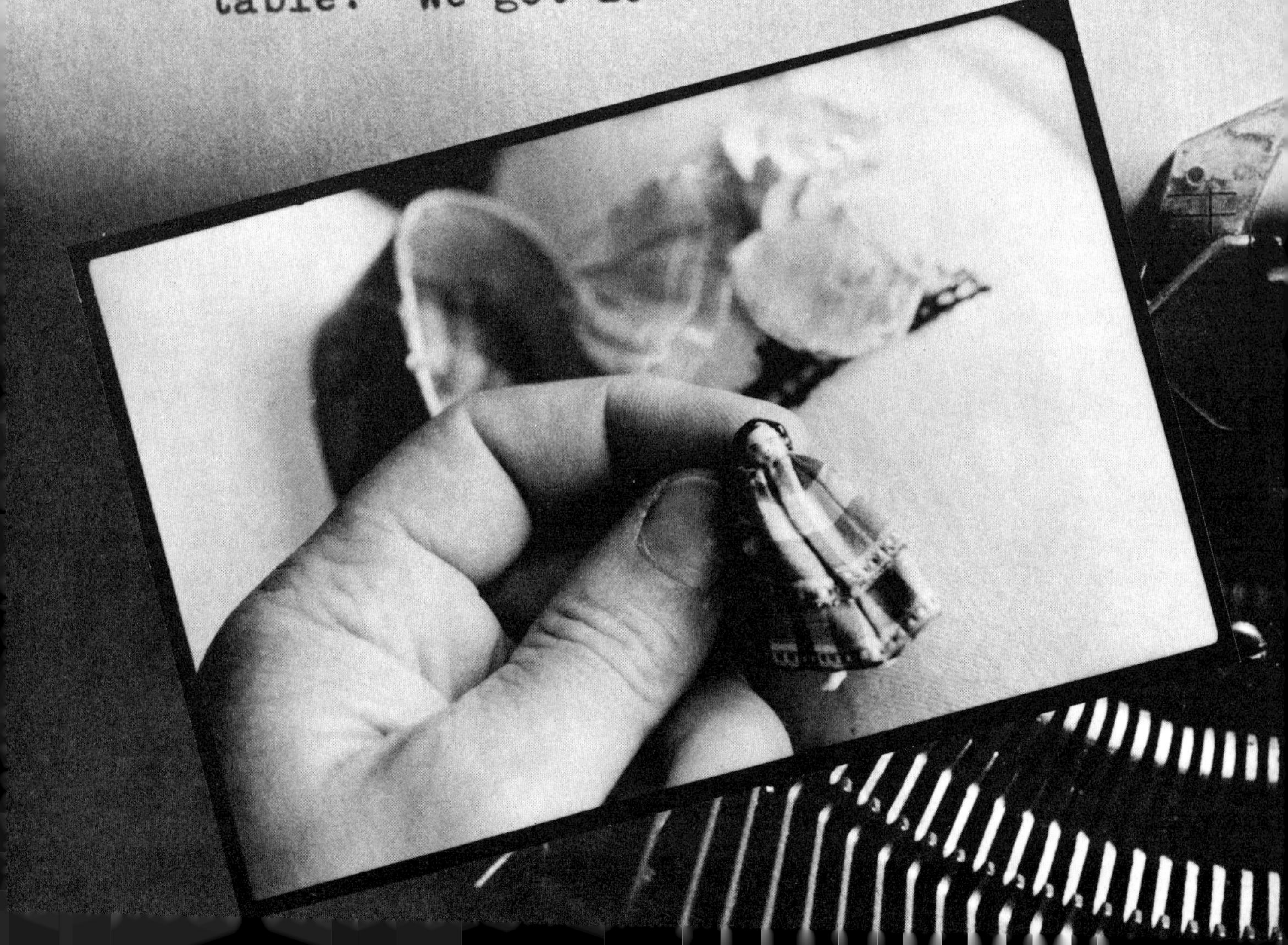

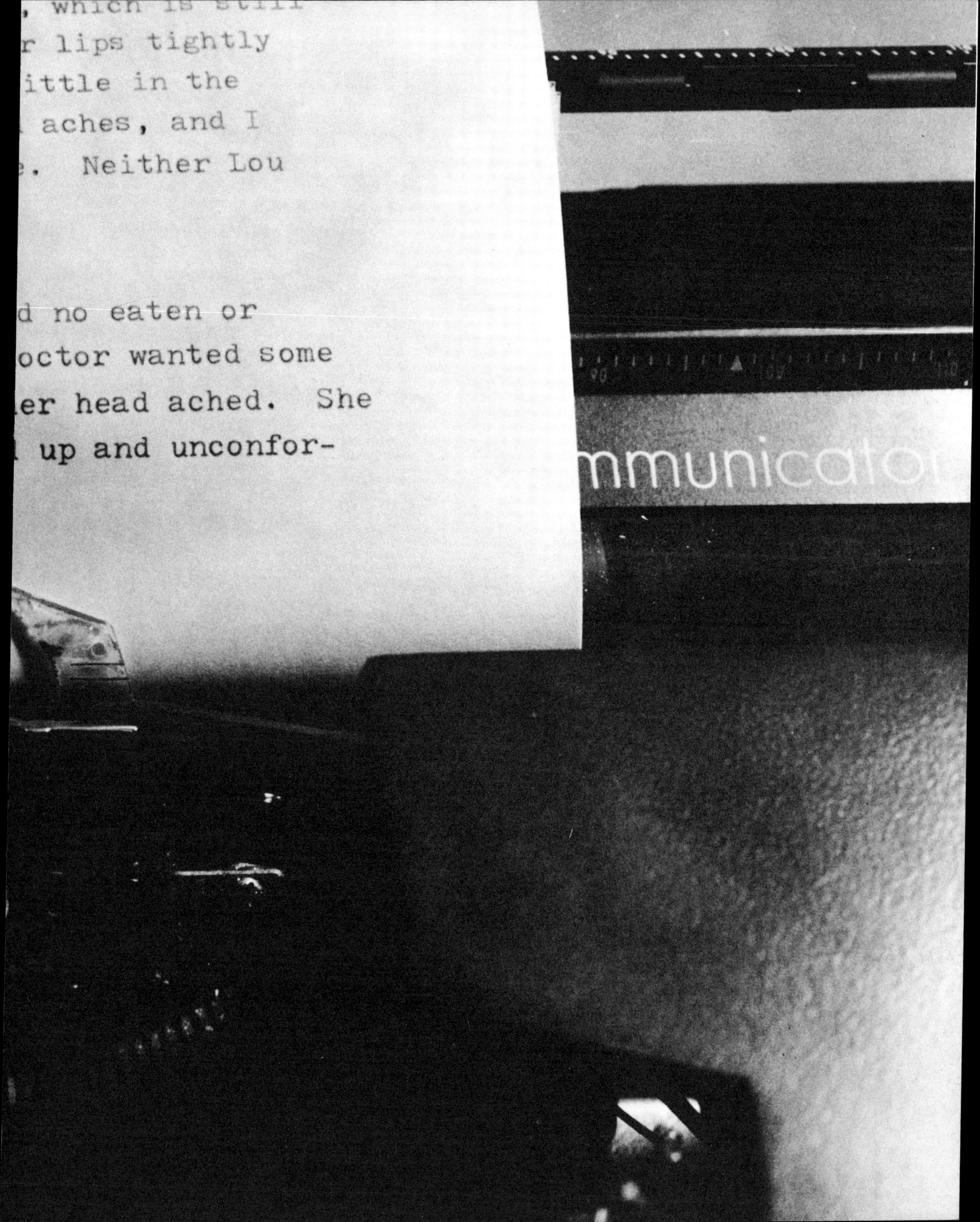

, which is
r lips tightly
ittle in the
aches, and I
. Neither Lou
d no eaten or
octor wanted some
er head ached. She
up and unconfor-
mmunicato

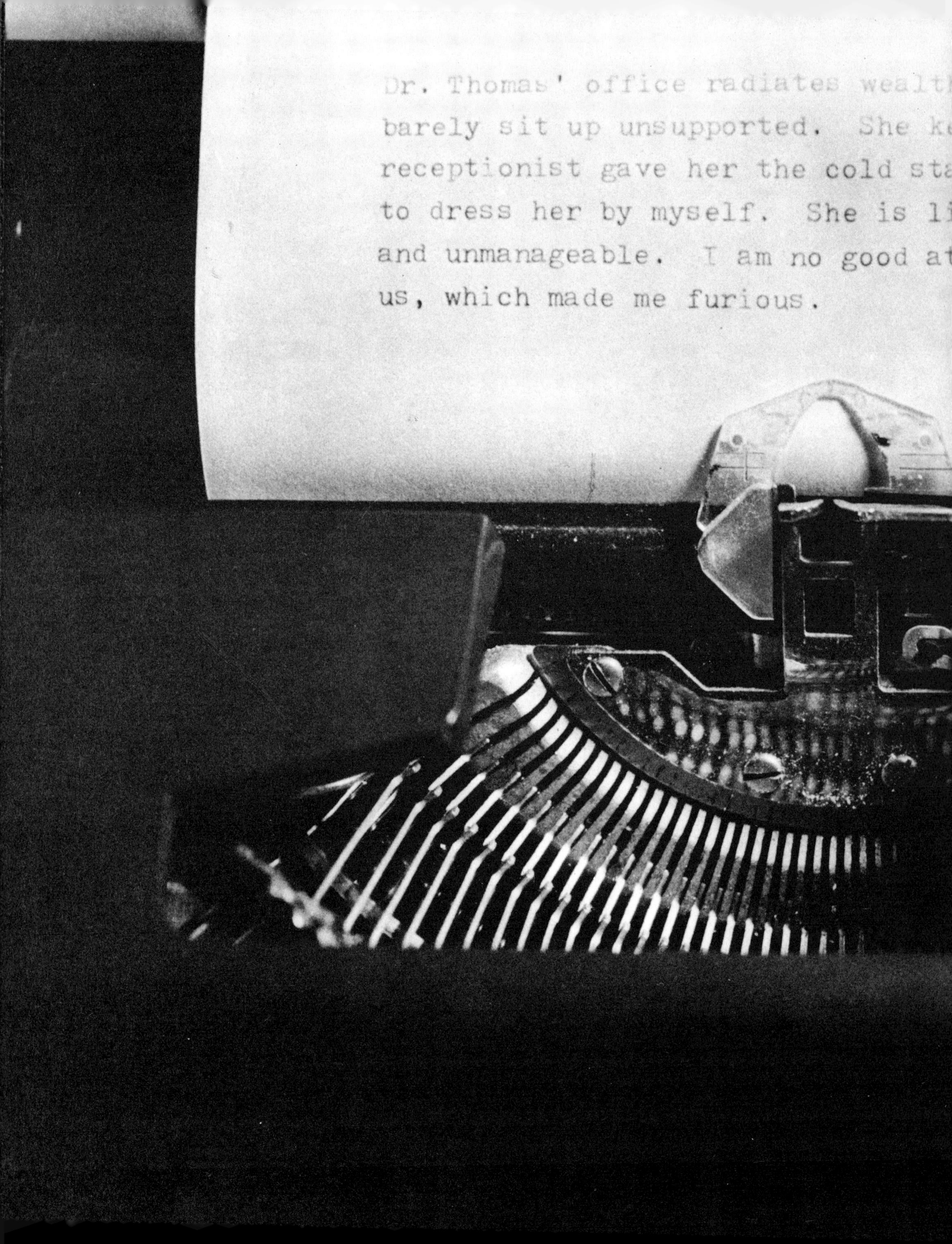
Dr. Thomas' office radiates
barely sit up unsupported. She
receptionist gave her the cold
to dress her by myself. She is
and unmanageable. I am no good
us, which made me furious.

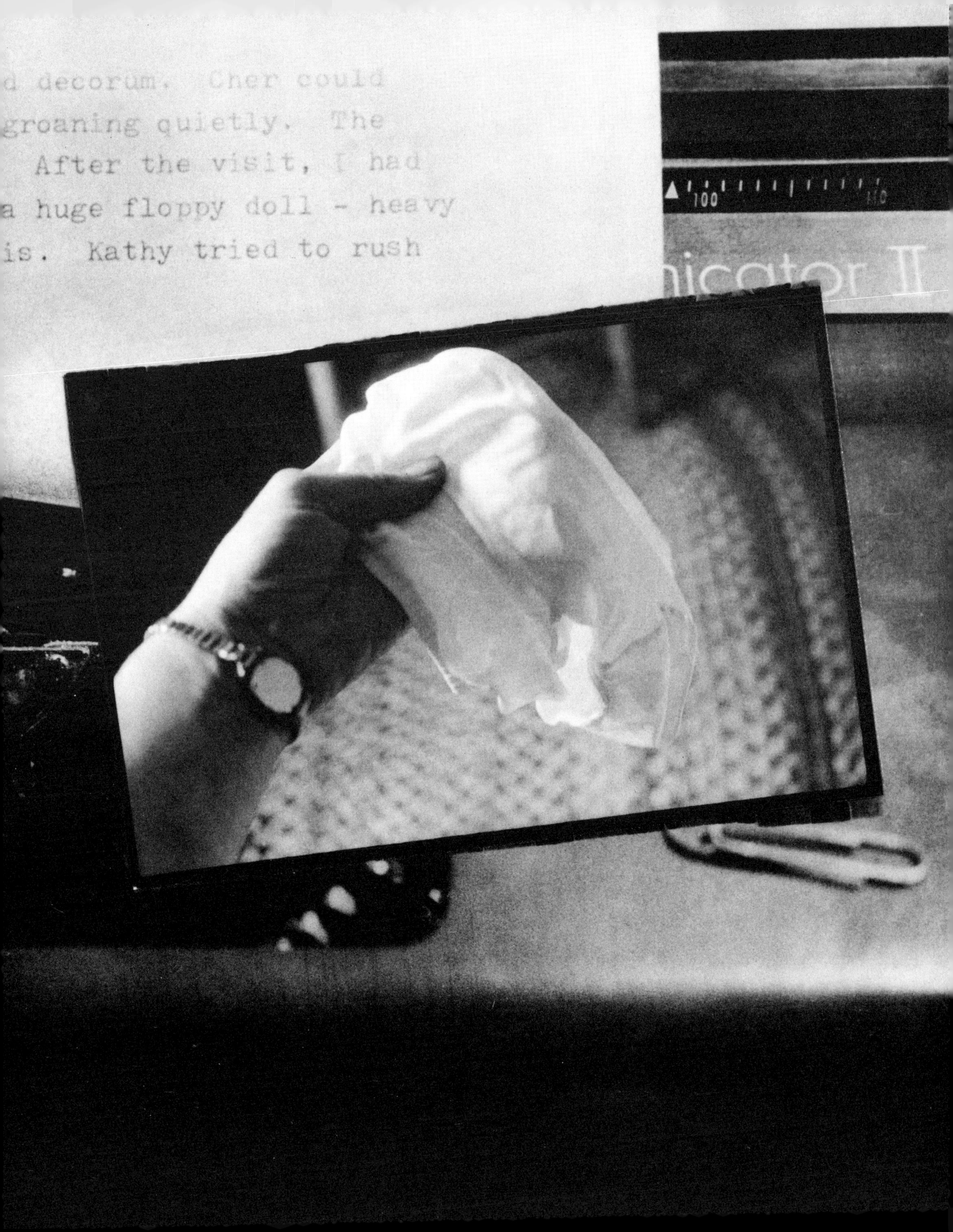
d decorum. Cher could
groaning quietly. The
After the visit, I had
a huge floppy doll - heavy
is. Kathy tried to rush
100
icator II

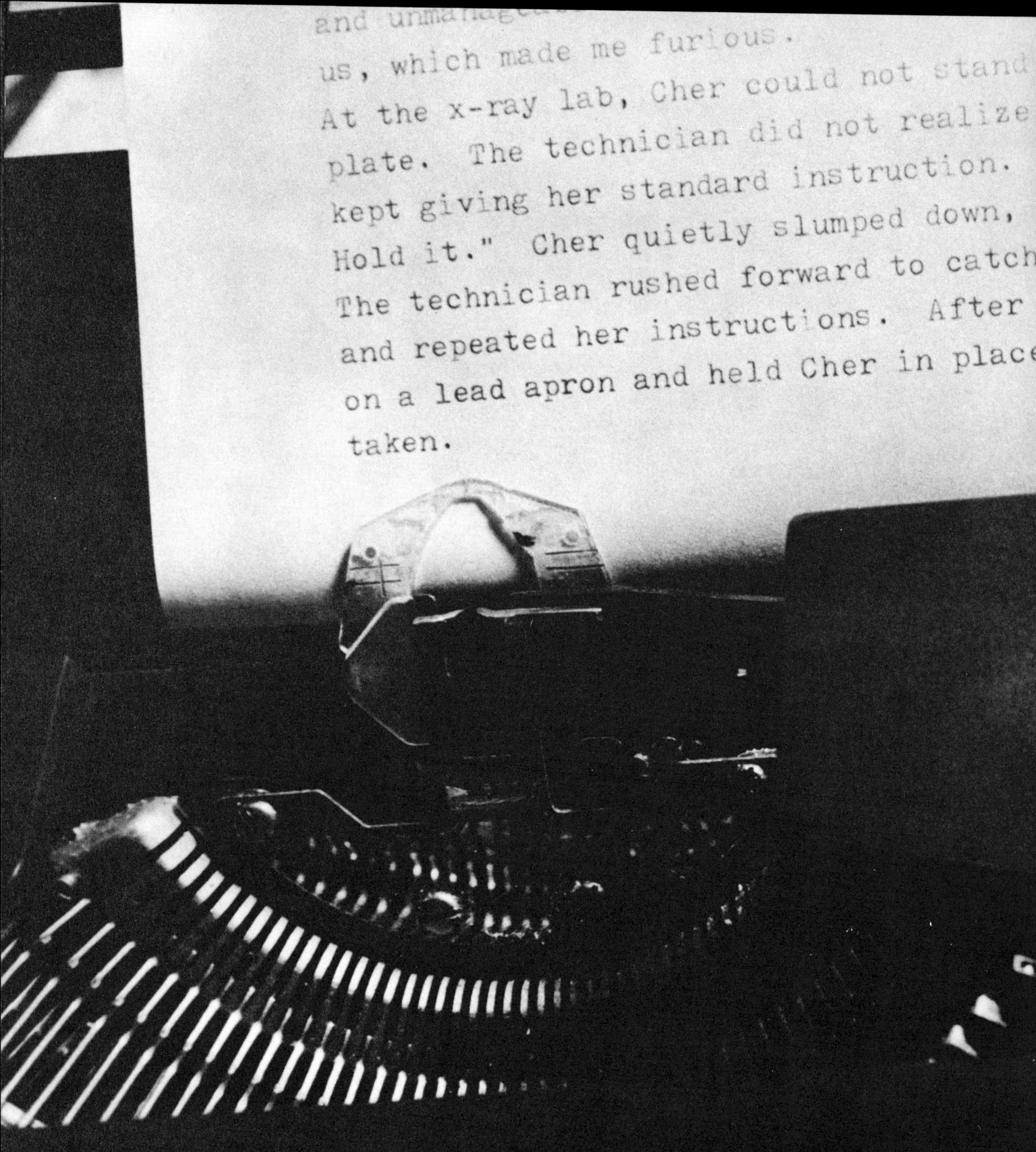
us, which made me furious.
At the x-ray lab, Cher could not stand
plate. The technician did not realize
kept giving her standard instruction.
Hold it." Cher quietly slumped down,
The technician rushed forward to
and repeated her instructions. After
on a lead apron and held Cher in
taken.

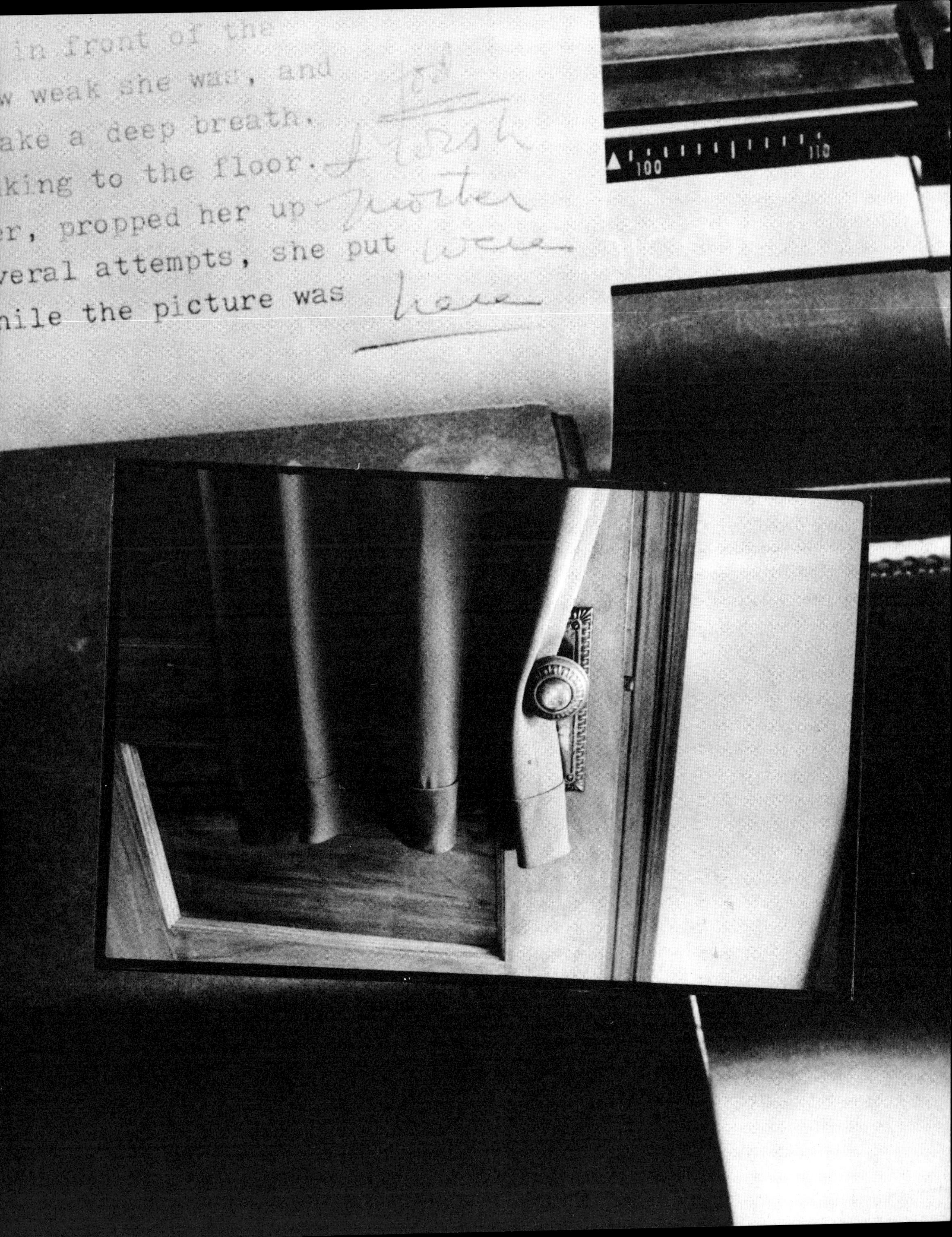
in front of the
w weak she was, and
ake a deep breath.
king to the floor.
er, propped her up
veral attempts, she put
hile the picture was
100
110

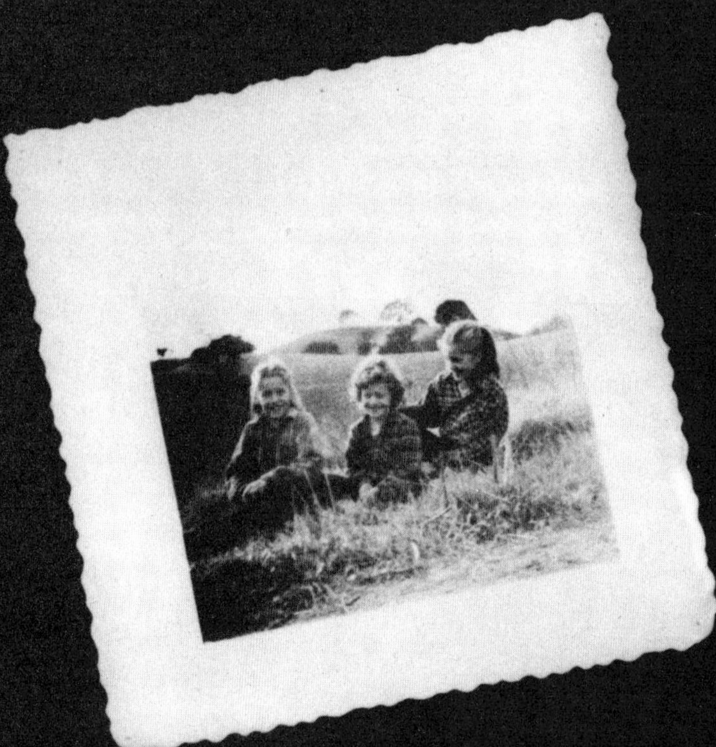

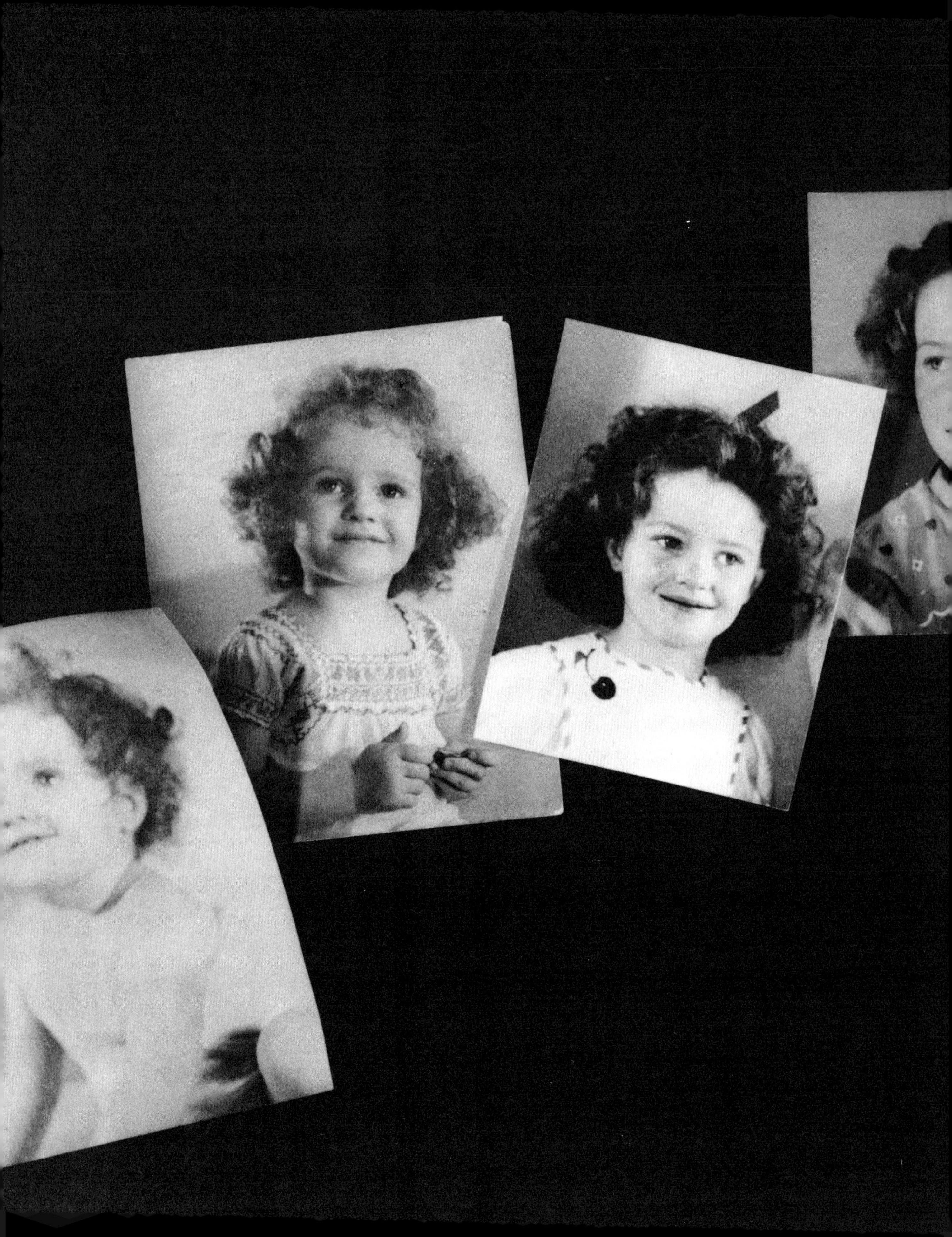

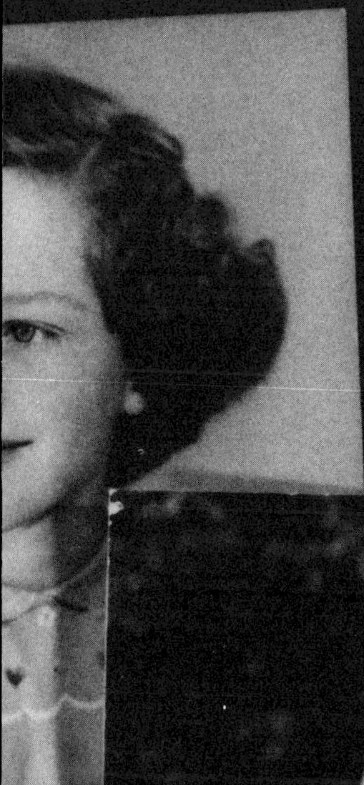
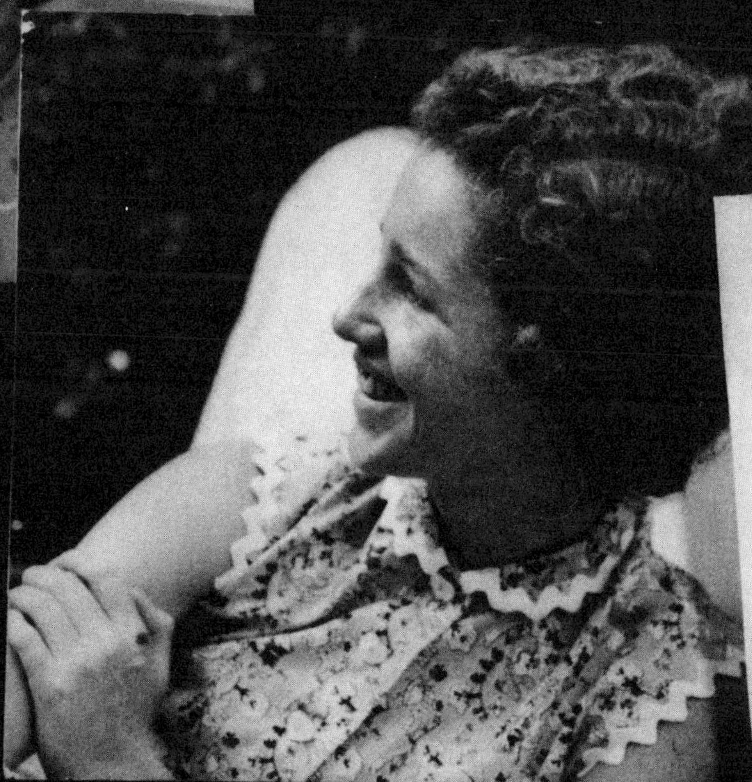
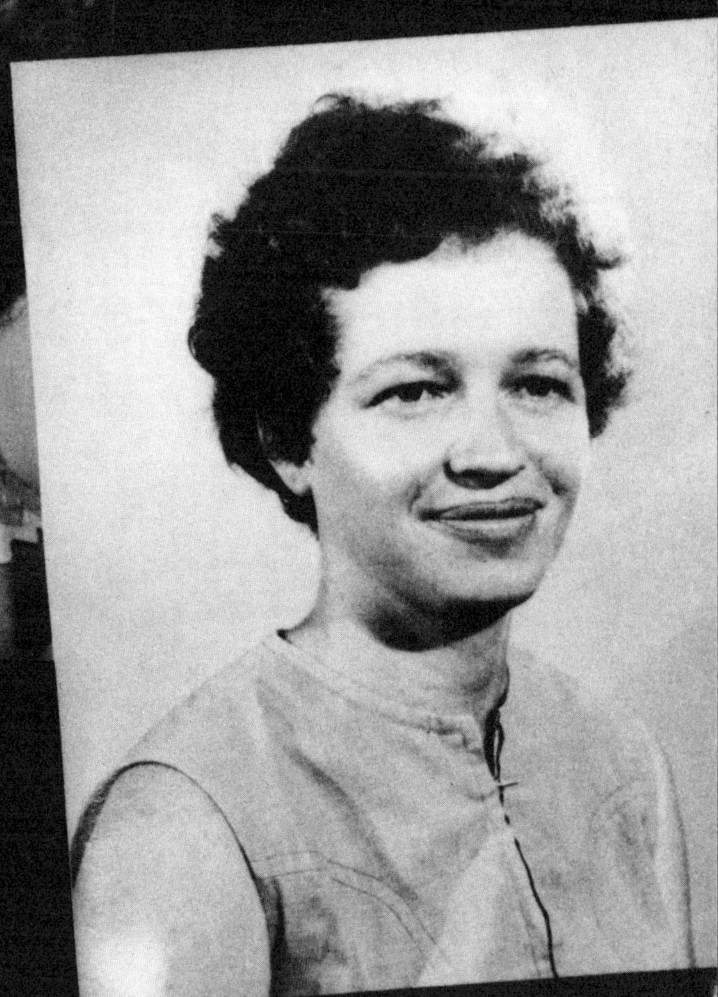

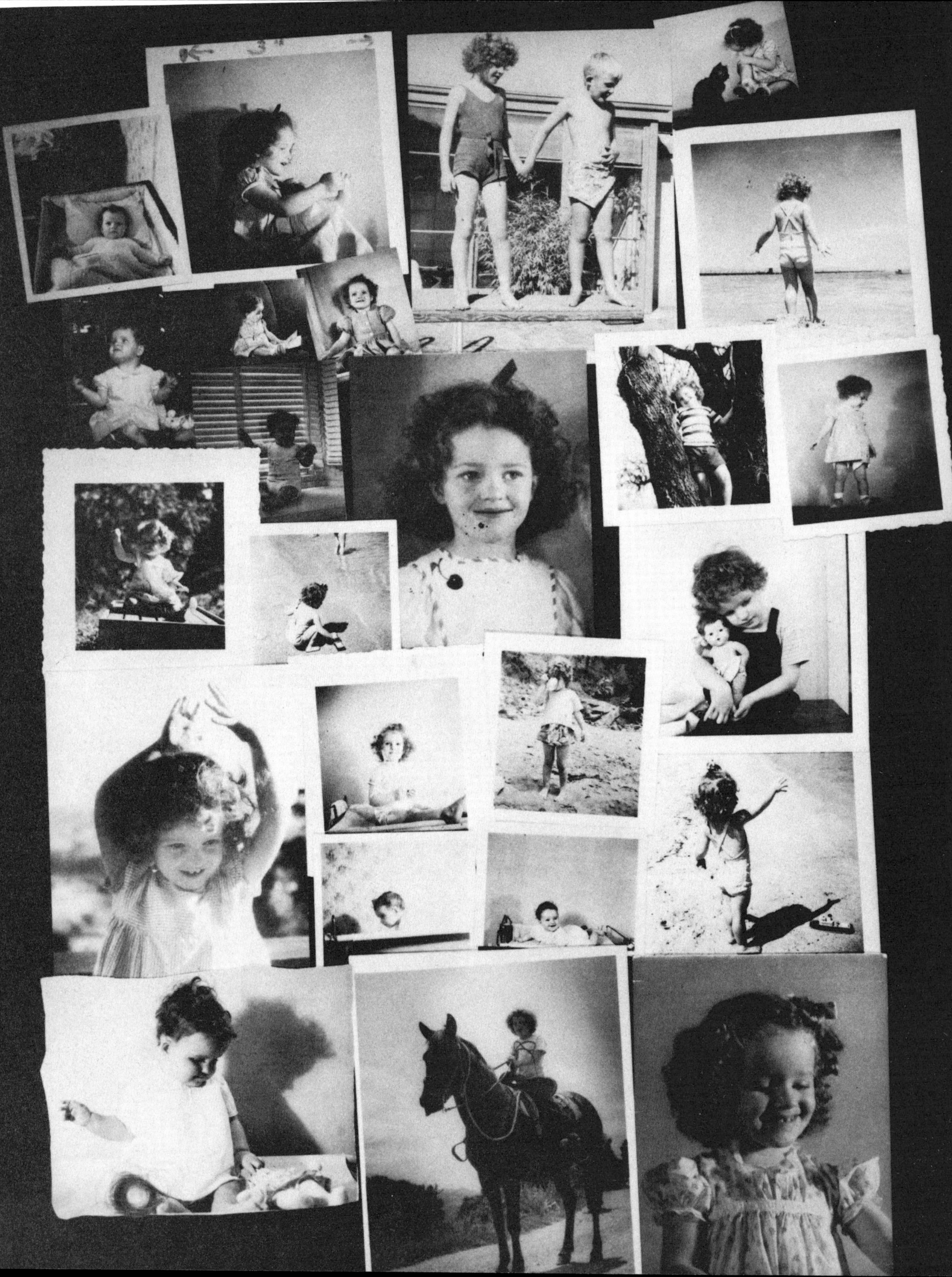

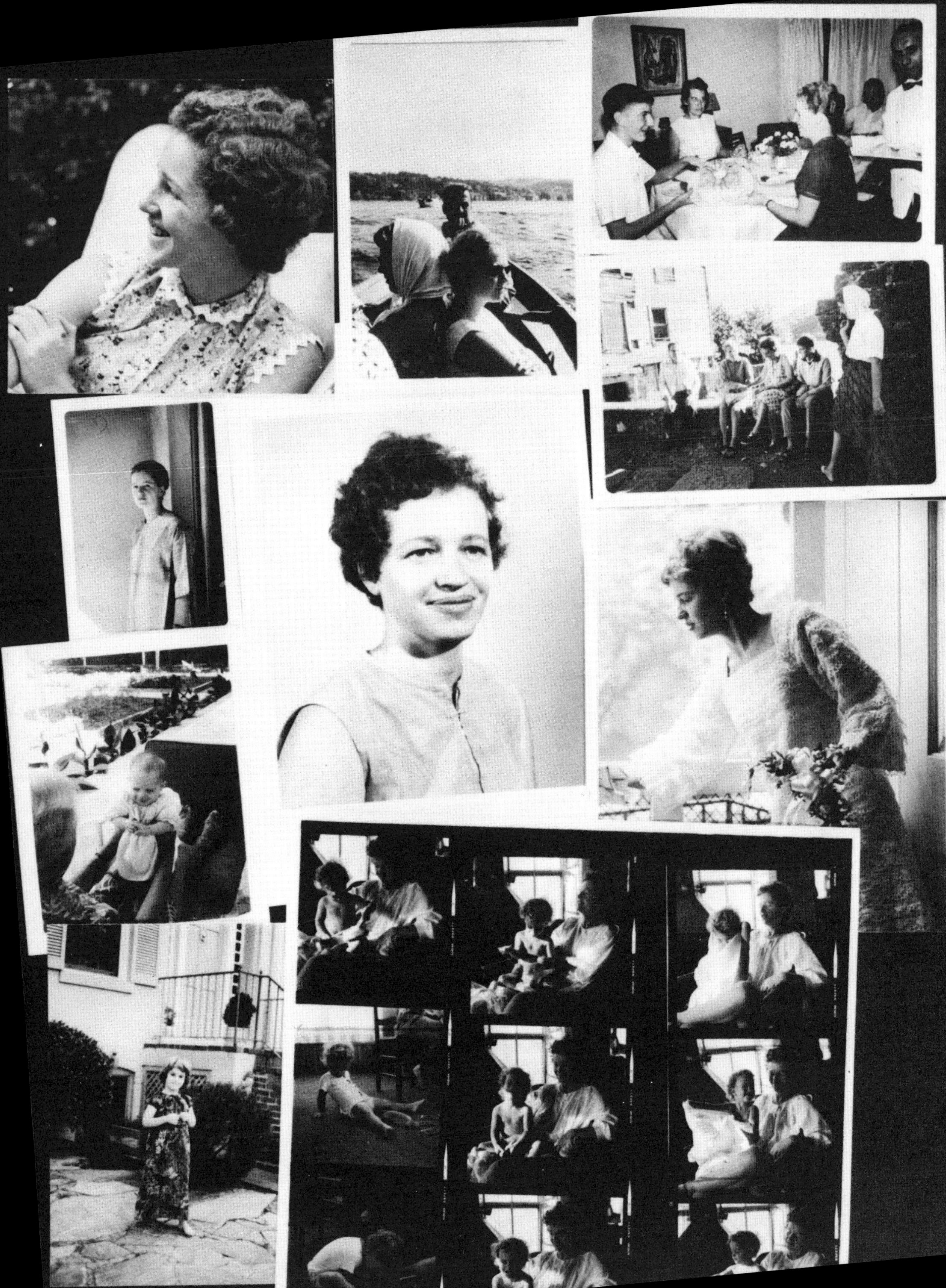

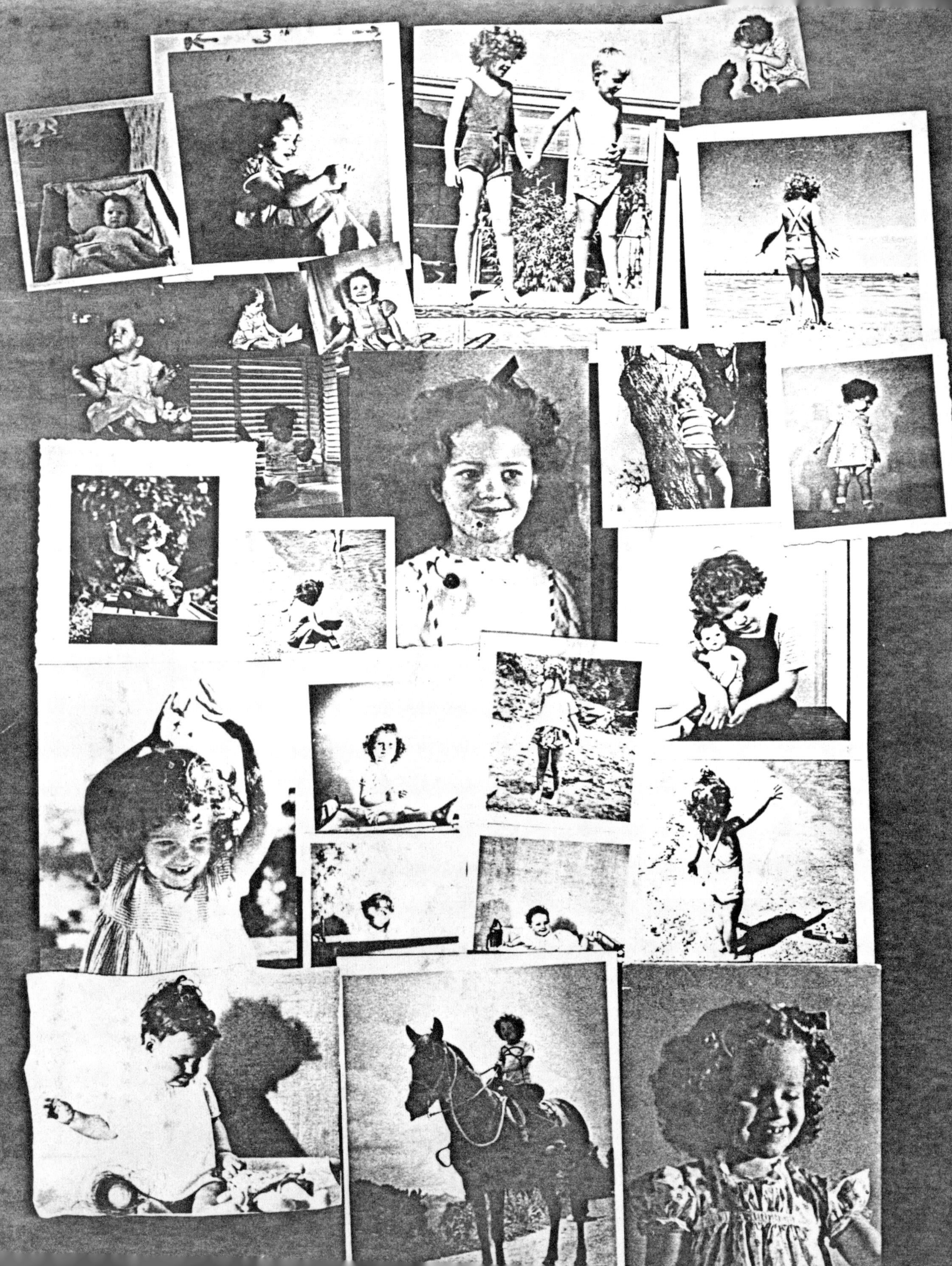

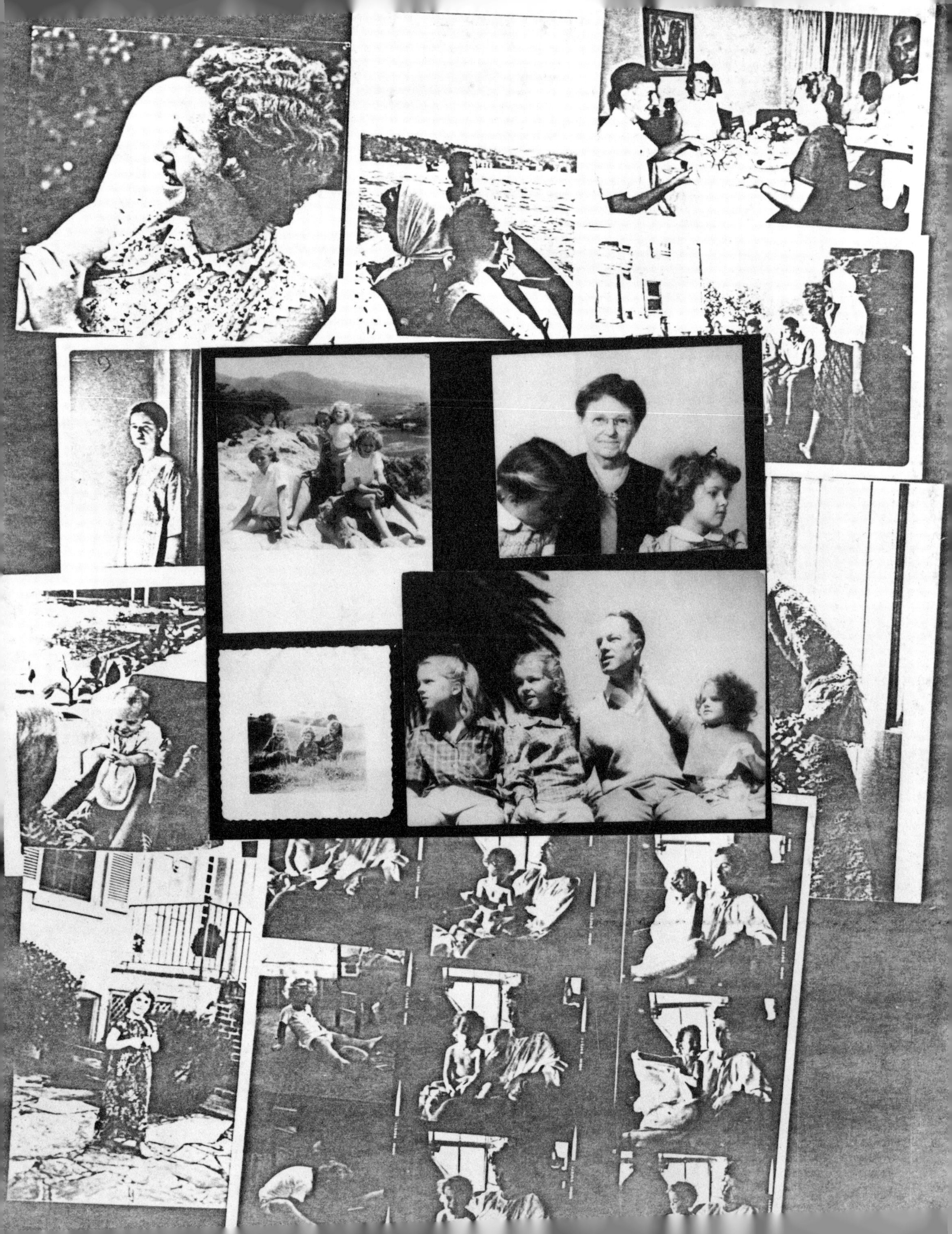

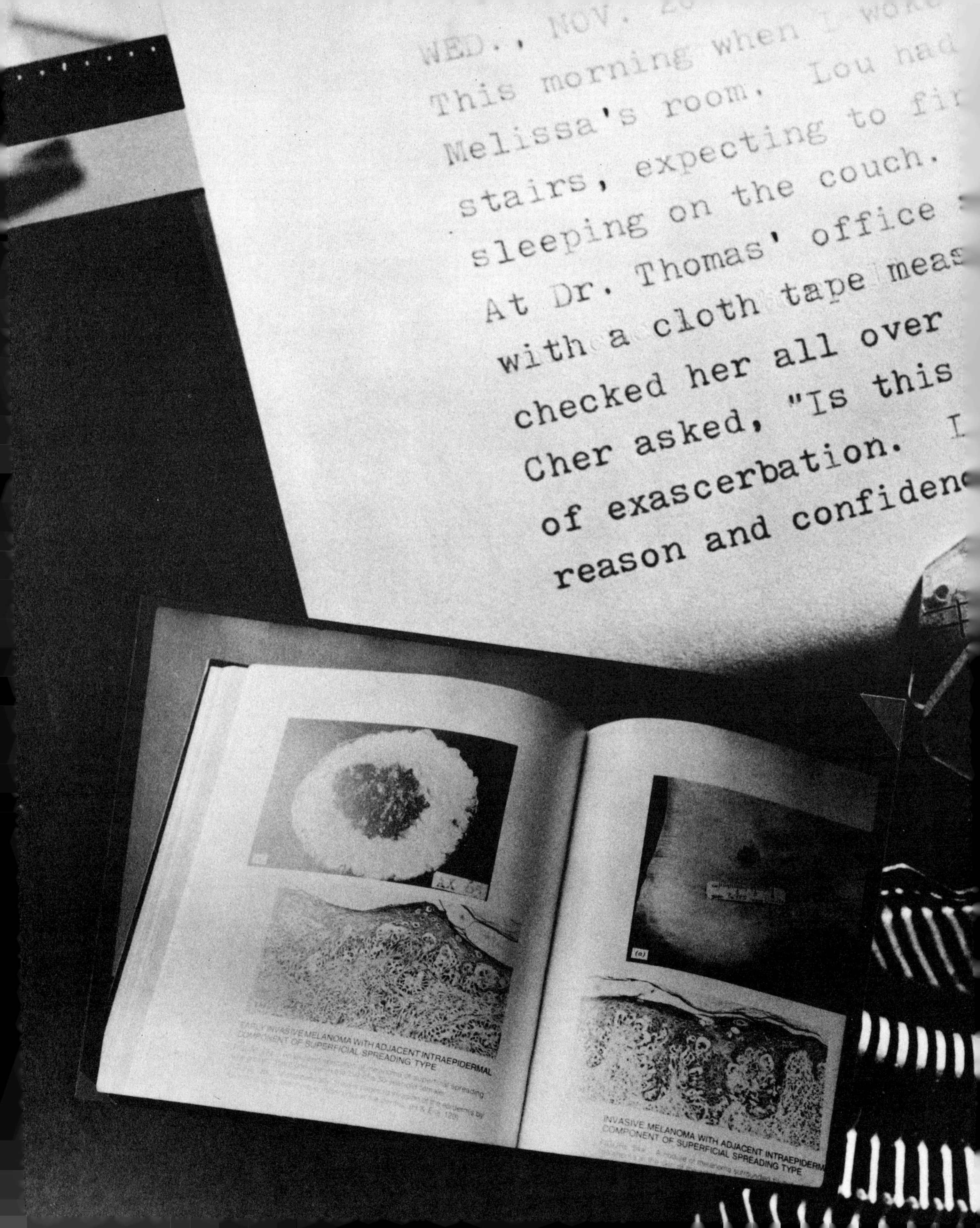
WED., NOV.
This morning when I
Melissa's room. Lou
stairs, expecting to
sleeping on the couch.
At Dr. Thomas' office
with a cloth tape
checked her all over
Cher asked, "Is this
of exascerbation.
reason and
EARLY INVASIVE MELANOMA WITH ADJACENT INTRAEPIDERMAL
COMPONENT OF SUPERFICIAL SPREADING TYPE
INVASIVE MELANOMA WITH ADJACENT INTRAEPIDERM
COMPONENT OF SUPERFICIAL SPREADING TYPE

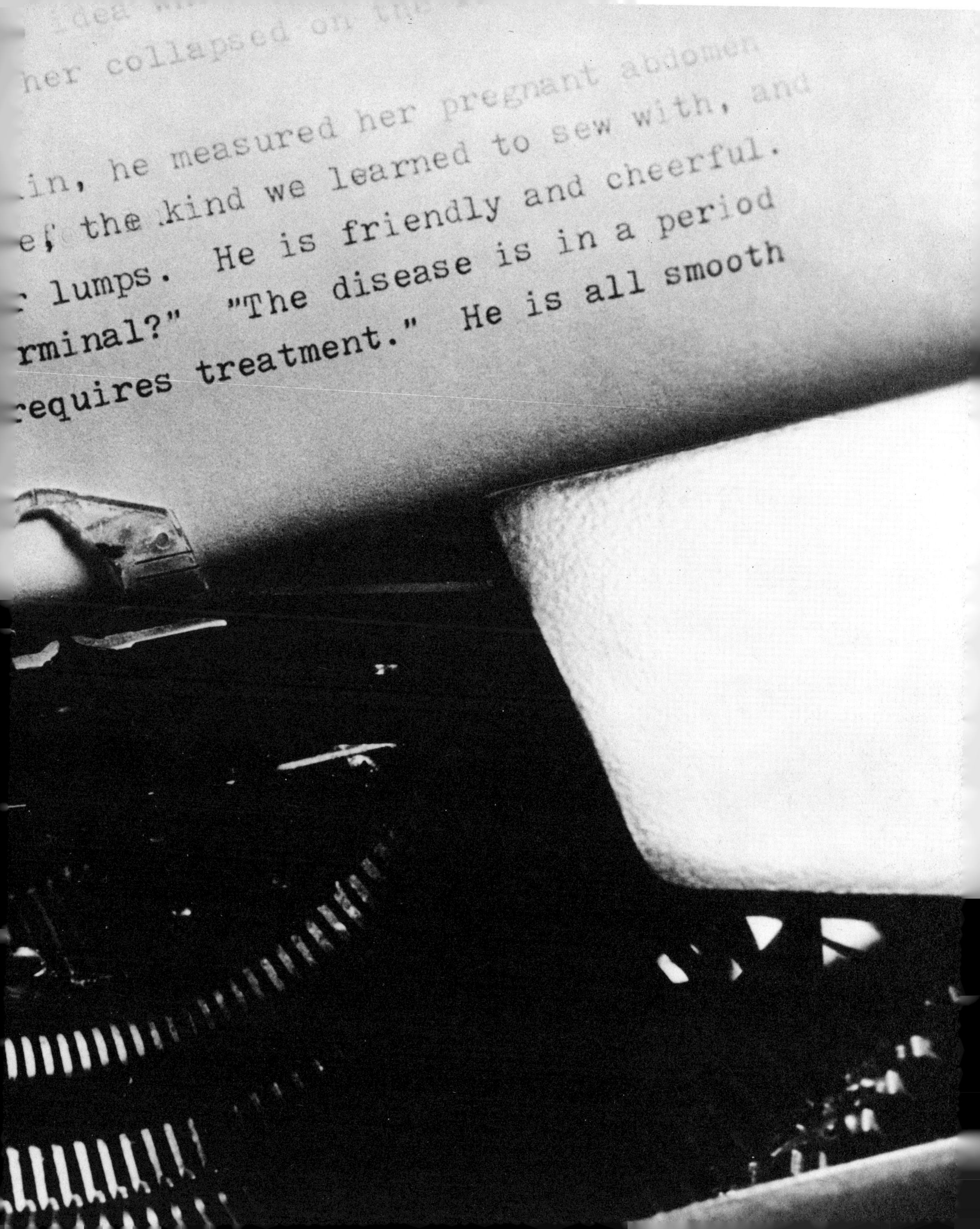
her collapsed on
in, he measured her pregnant abdomen
the kind we learned to sew with, and
lumps. He is friendly and cheerful.
rminal?" "The disease is in a period
requires treatment." He is all smooth

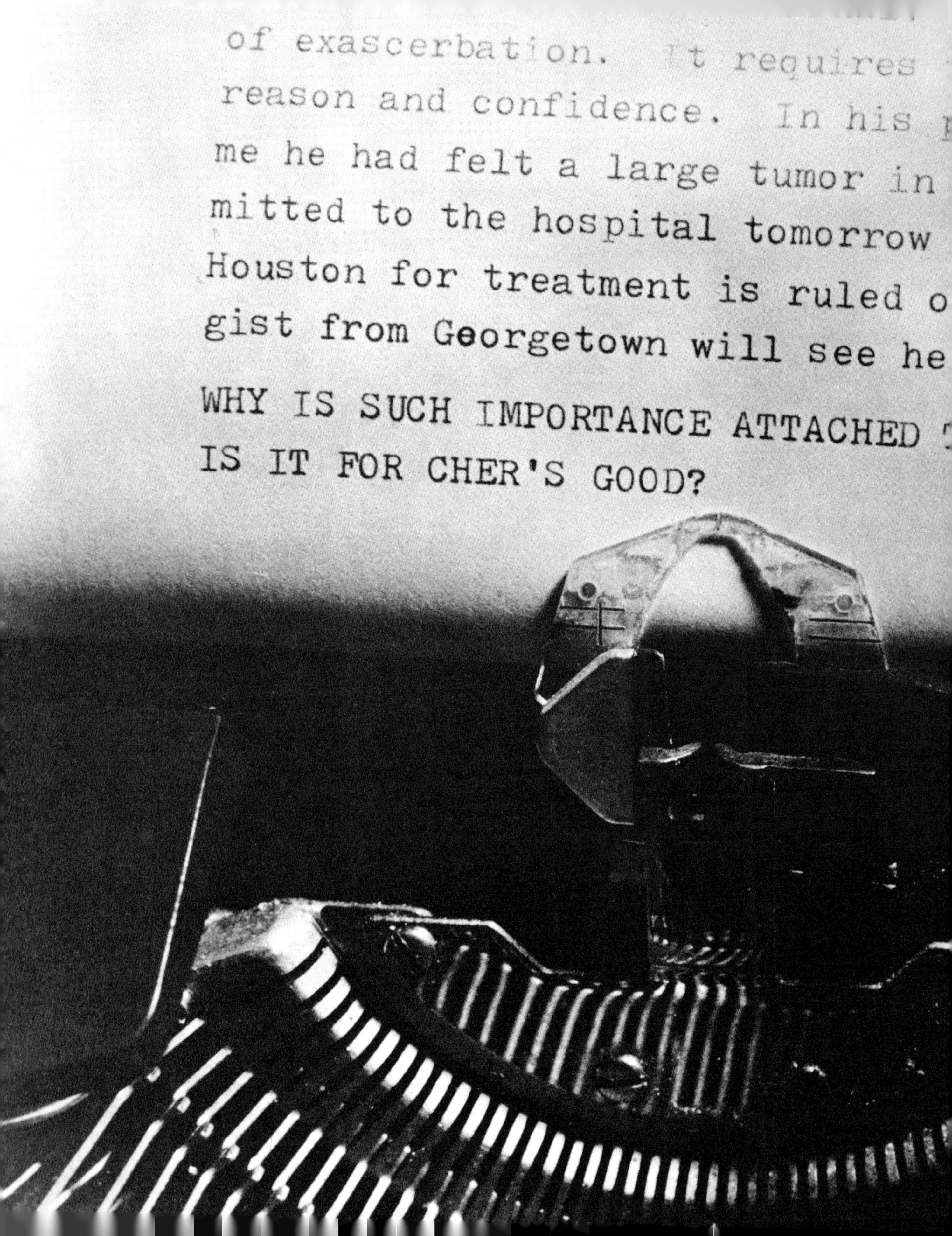
of exascerbation. It requires
reason and confidence. In his
me he had felt a large tumor in
mitted to the hospital tomorrow
Houston for treatment is ruled o
gist from Georgetown will see he
WHY IS SUCH IMPORTANCE ATTACHED
IS IT FOR CHER'S GOOD?

atment." He is all smooth
vate office, he told Lou and
r abdomen. She must be ad-
r an abortion. Travel to
for the moment. The oncolo-
next week.

PERFORMING THIS ABORTION?

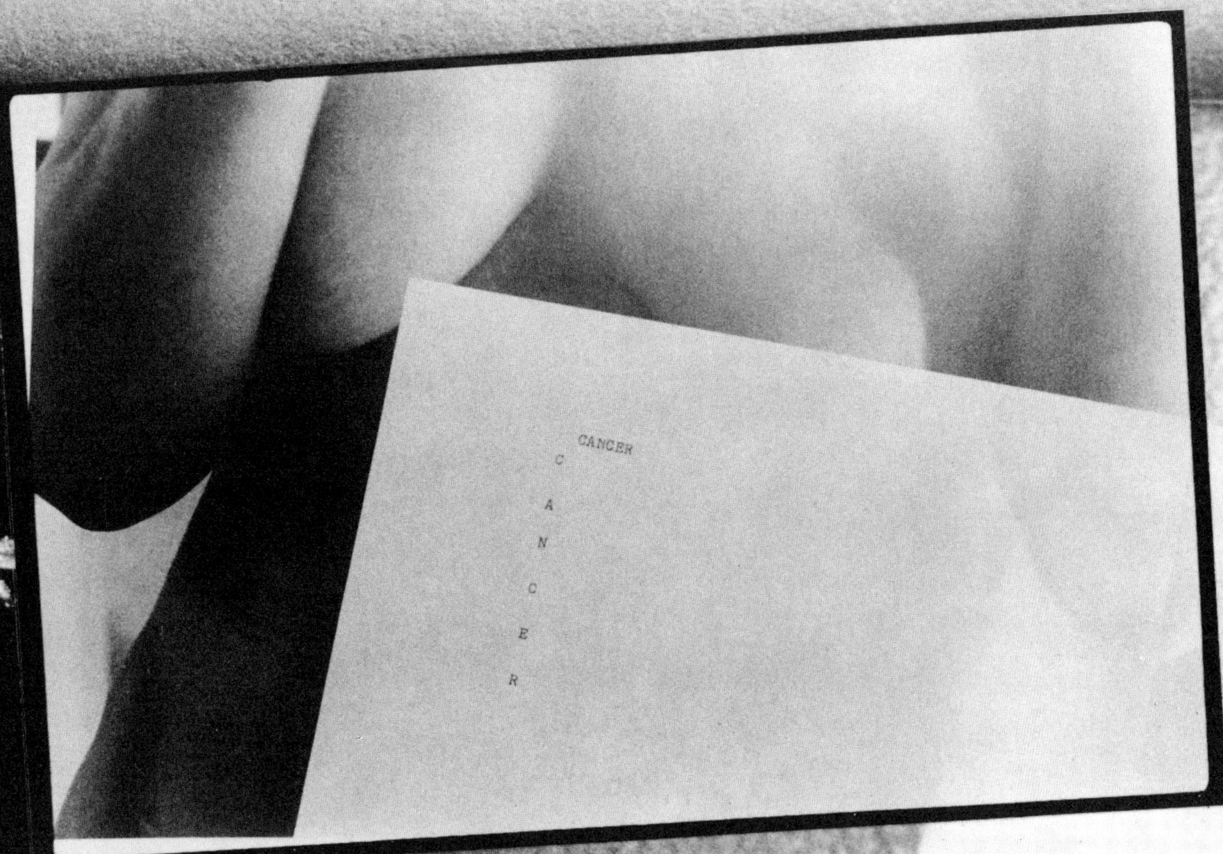

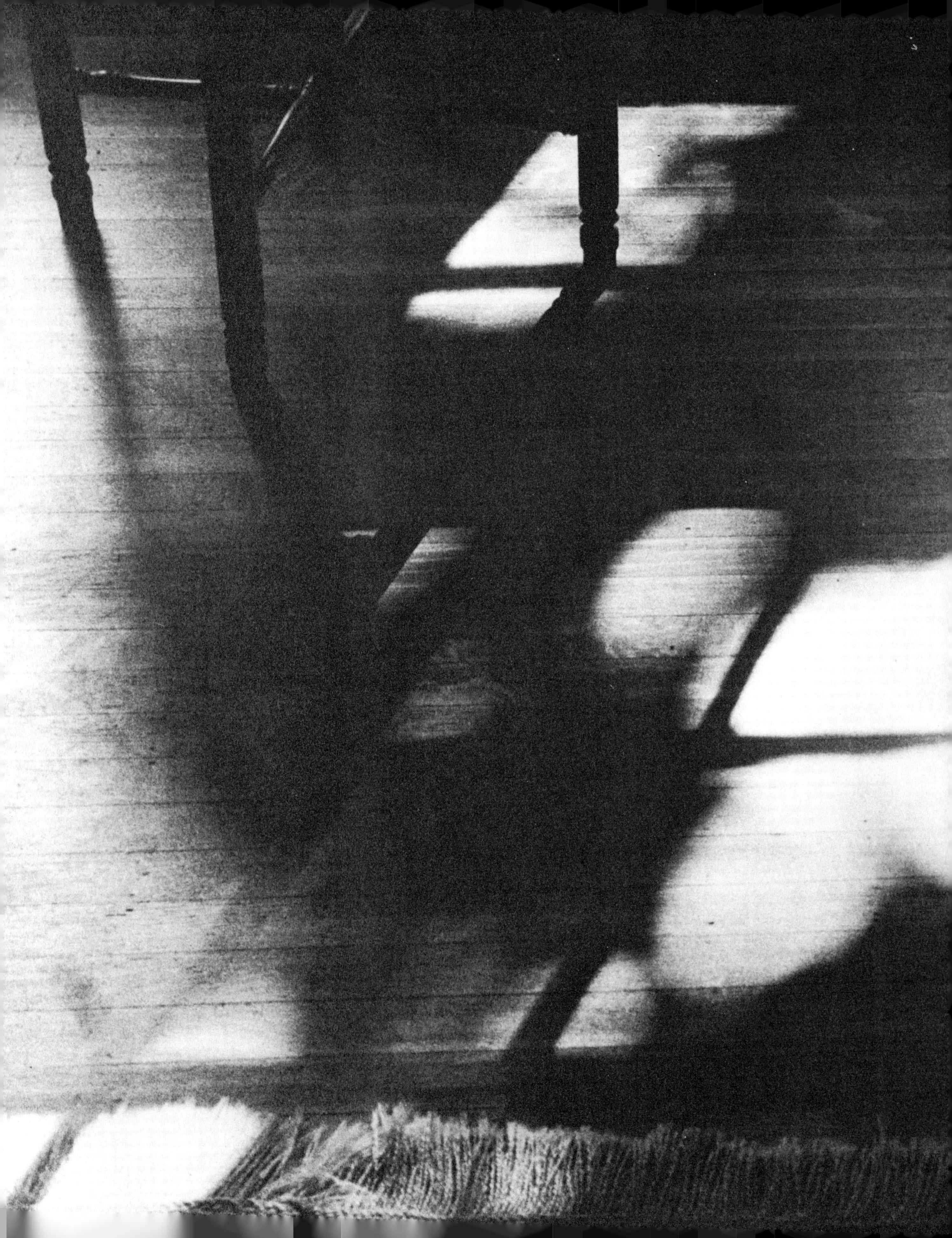

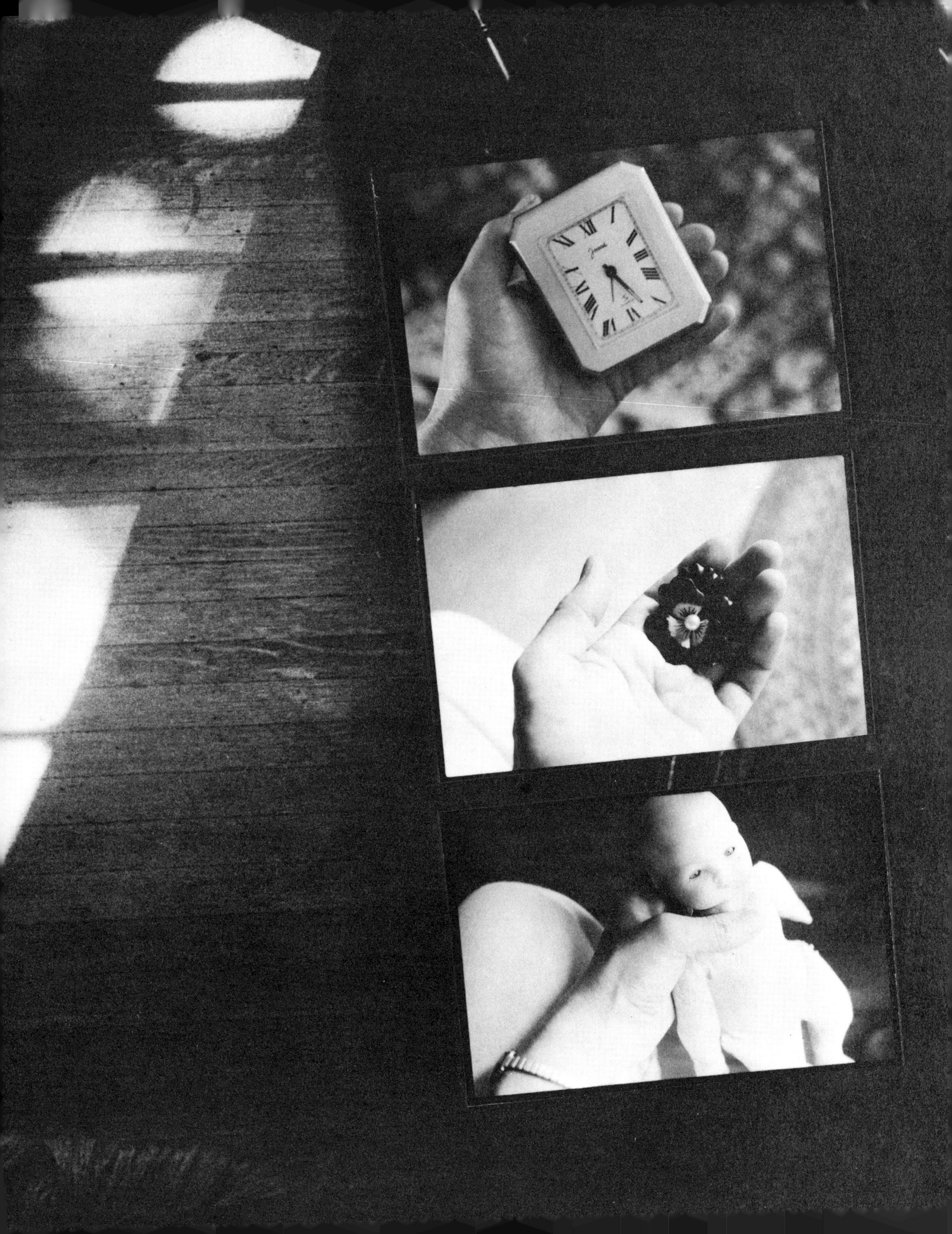

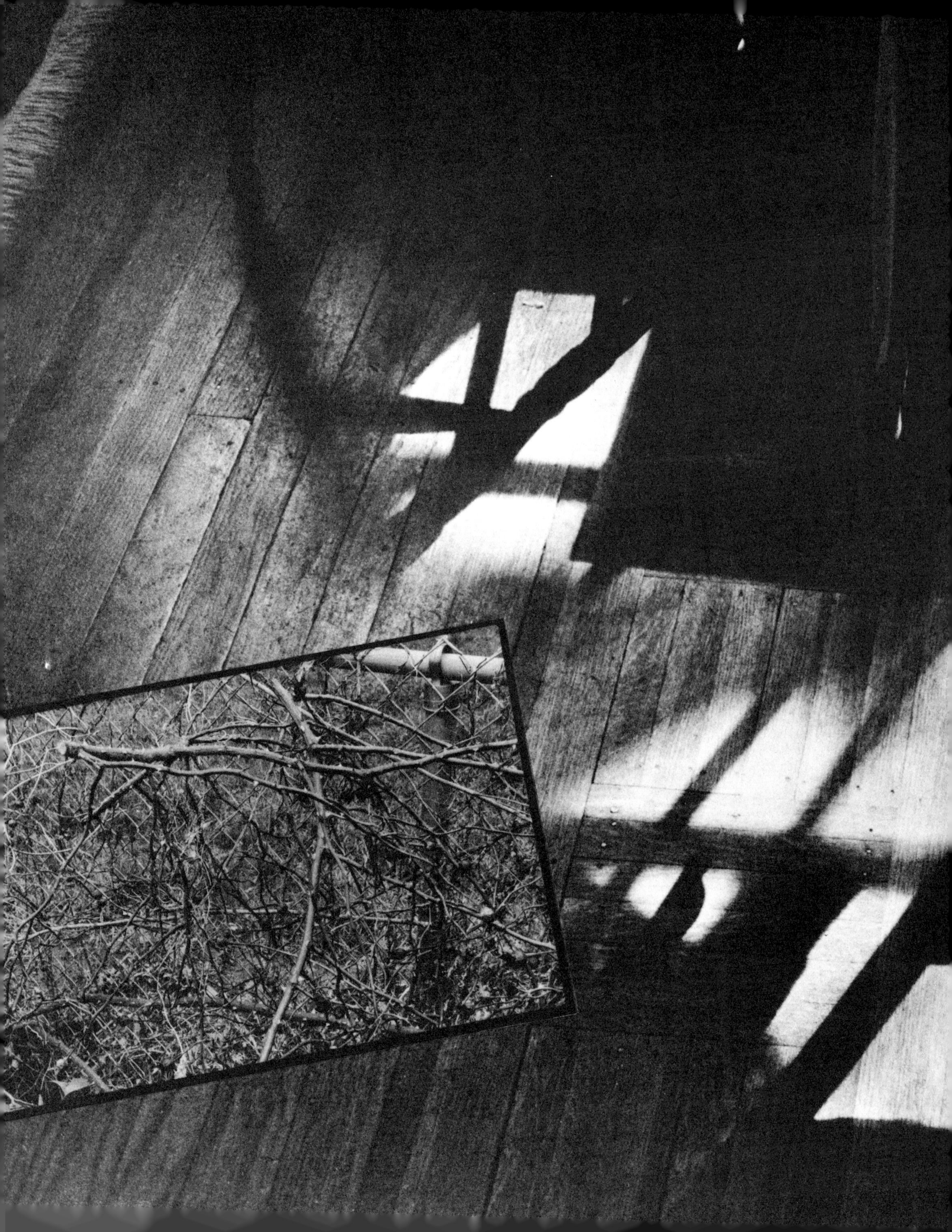

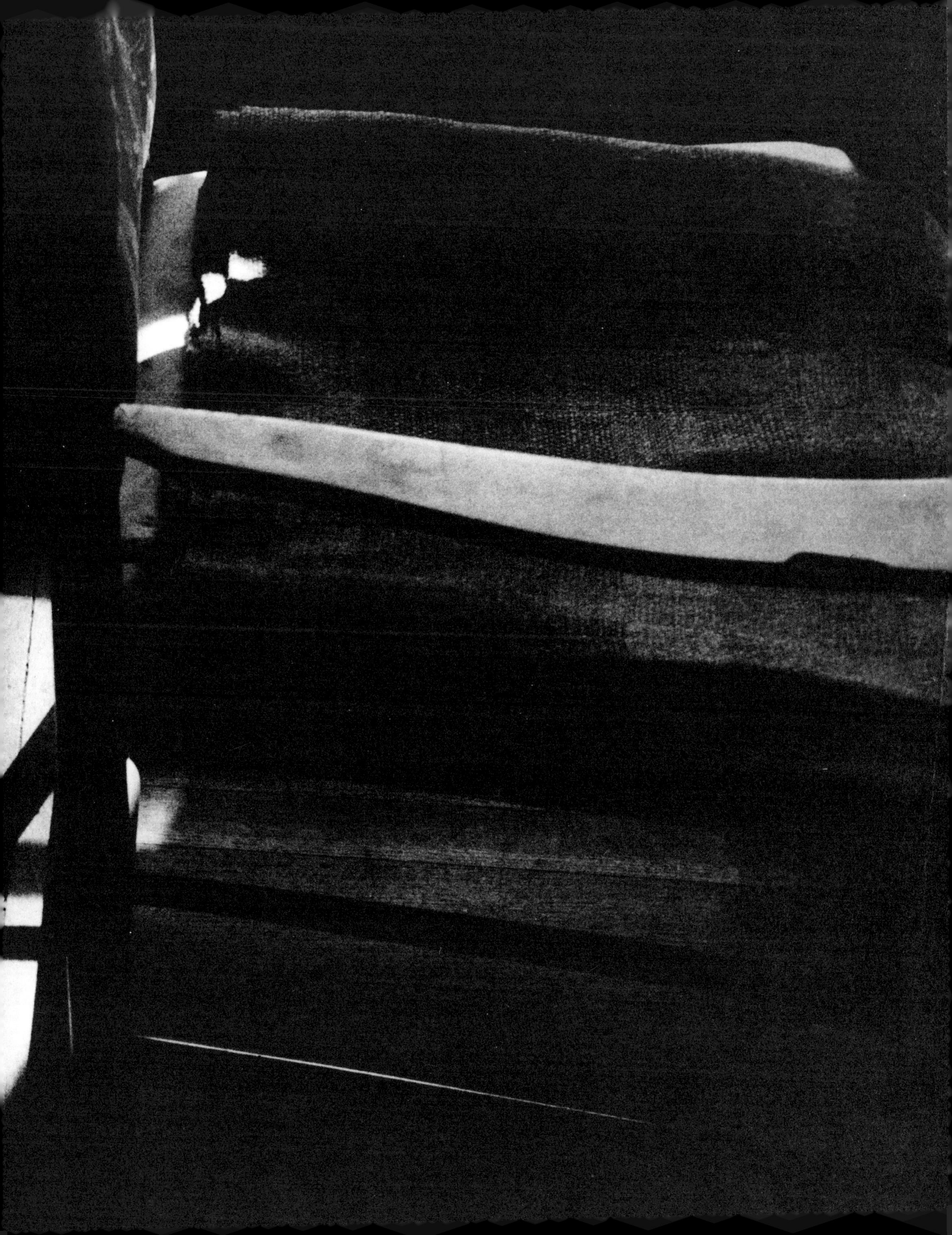

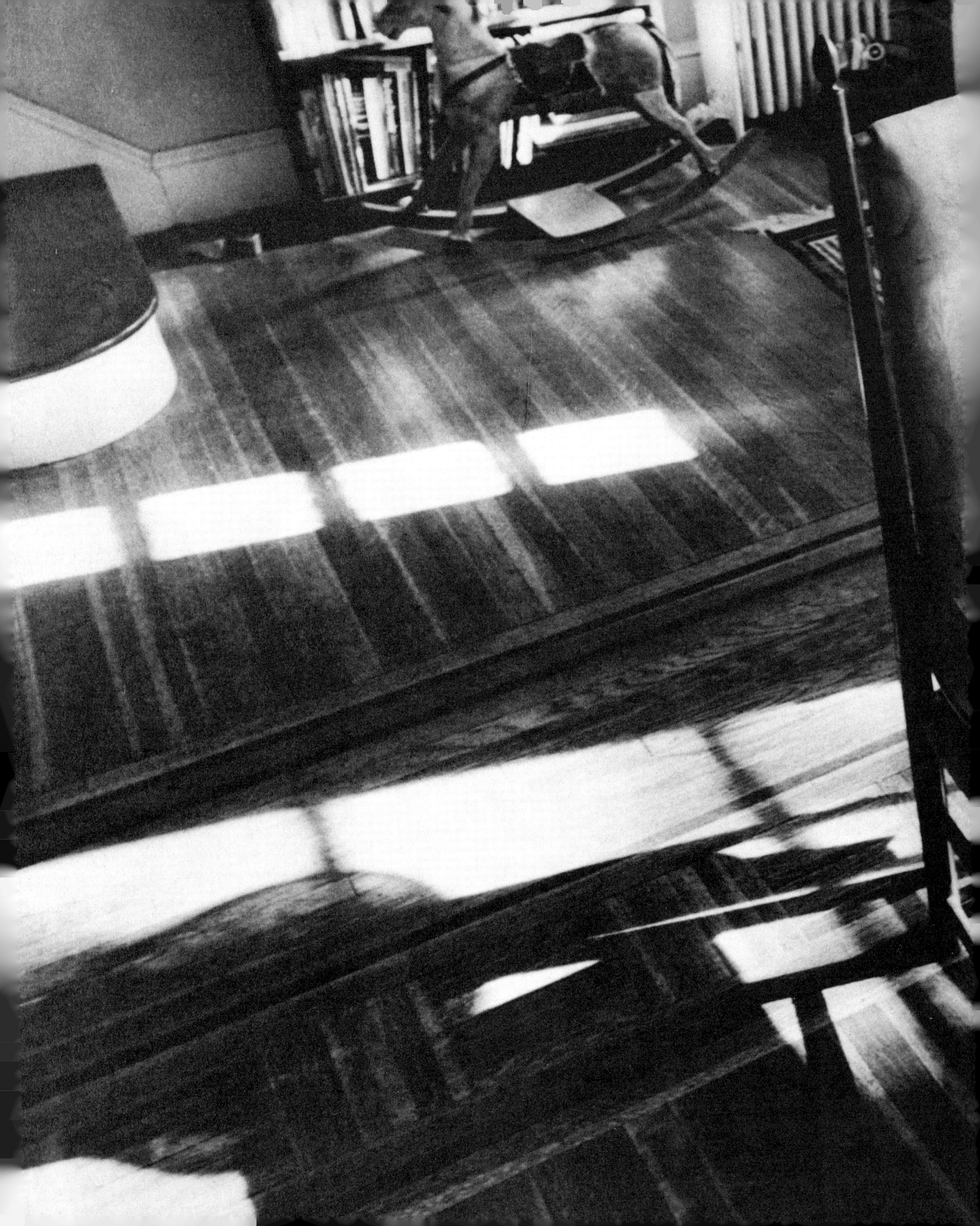

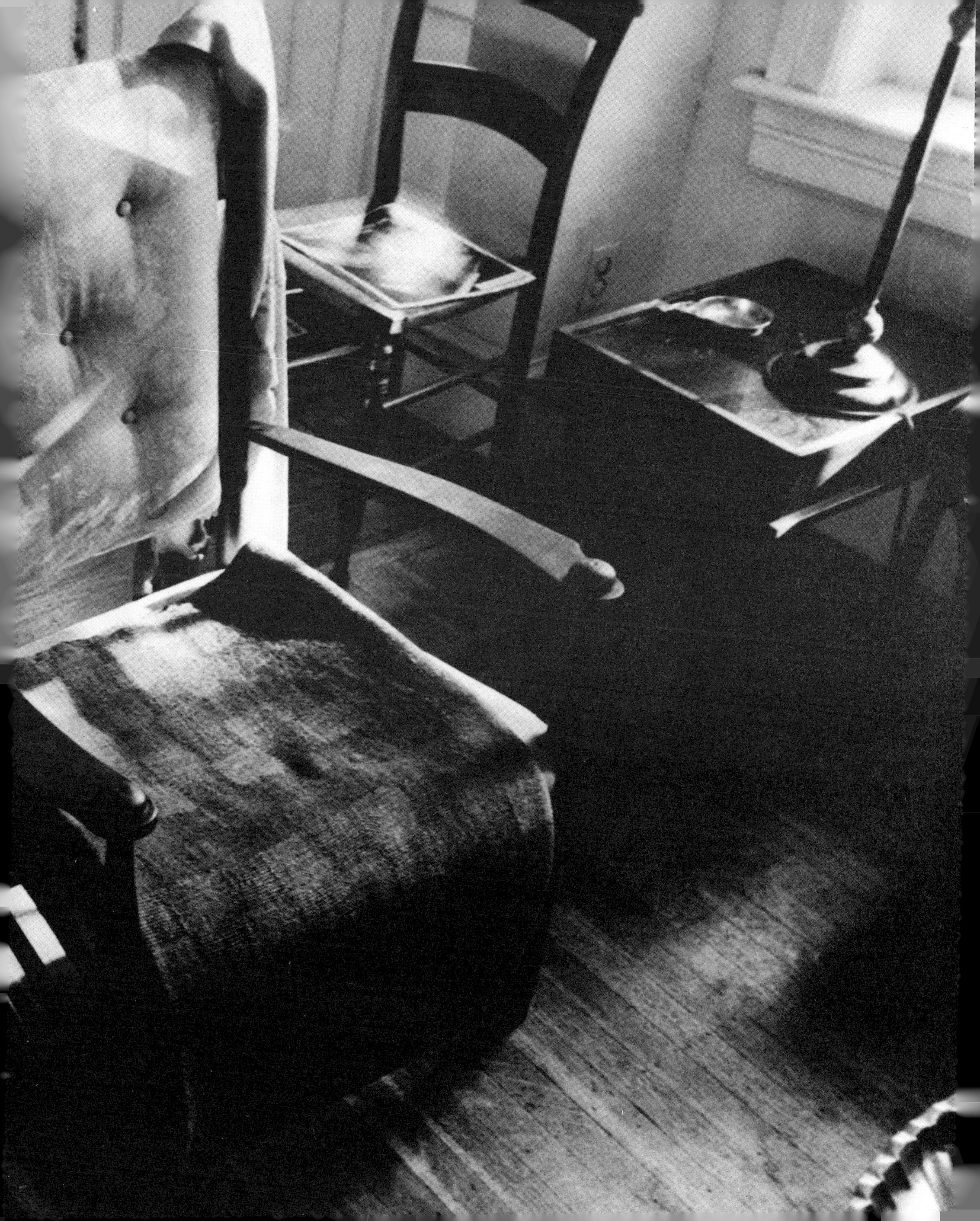

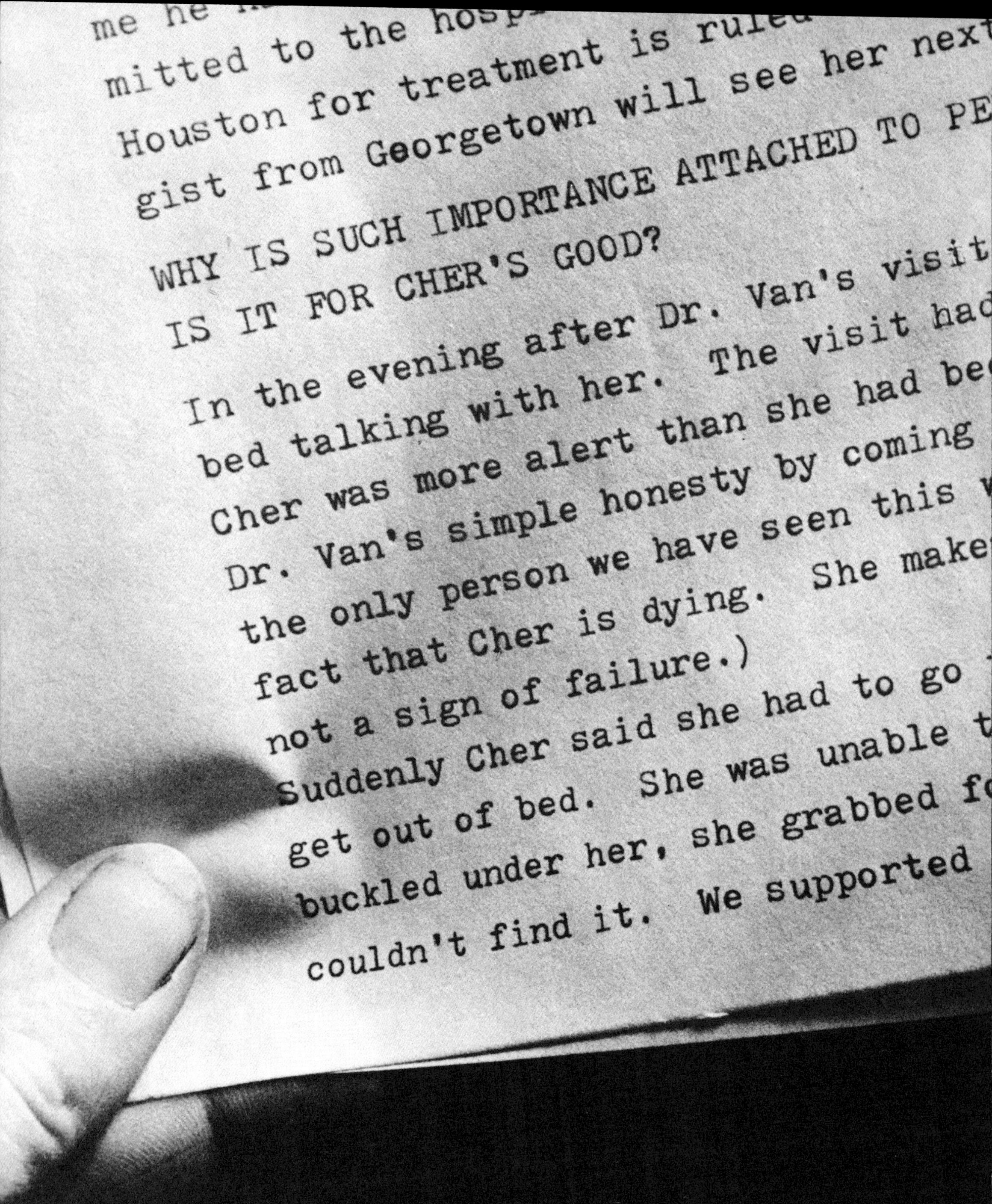
me he
mitted to the hosp
Houston for treatment is rule
gist from Georgetown will see her next
WHY IS SUCH IMPORTANCE ATTACHED TO PE
IS IT FOR CHER'S GOOD?
In the evening after Dr. Van's visit
bed talking with her. The visit had
Cher was more alert than she had be
Dr. Van's simple honesty by coming
the only person we have seen this
fact that Cher is dying. She make
not a sign of failure.)
Suddenly Cher said she had to go
get out of bed. She was unable t
buckled under her, she grabbed f
couldn't find it. We supported

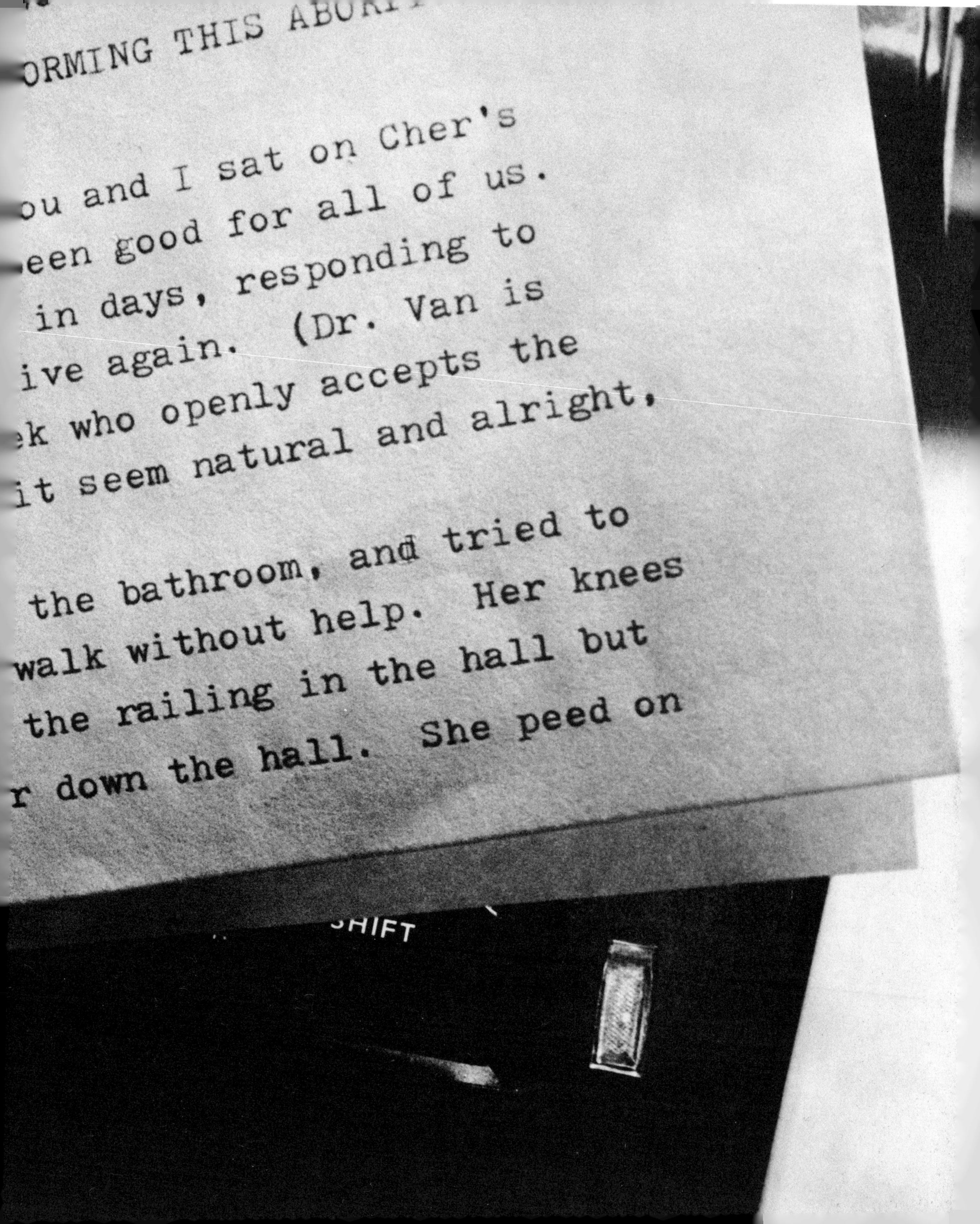
ORMING THIS ABORT
ou and I sat on Cher's
een good for all of us.
in days, responding to
ive again. (Dr. Van is
ek who openly accepts the
it seem natural and alright,
the bathroom, and tried to
walk without help. Her knees
the railing in the hall but
r down the hall. She peed on
SHIFT

the floor before reaching the bathro
was doing.
It is appalling to me how fast she is
yesterday she took a shower and washe
I thought it wrong to intrude on her
independence by checking to make sure

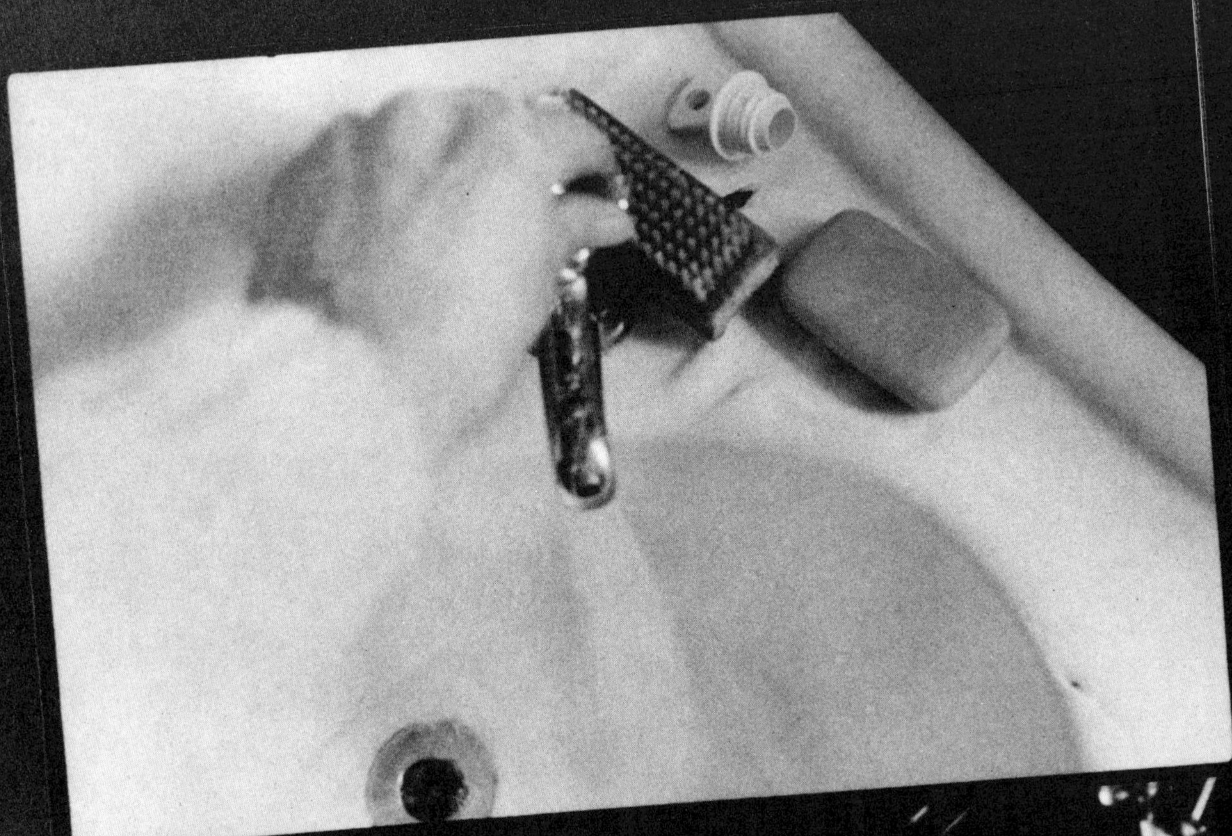

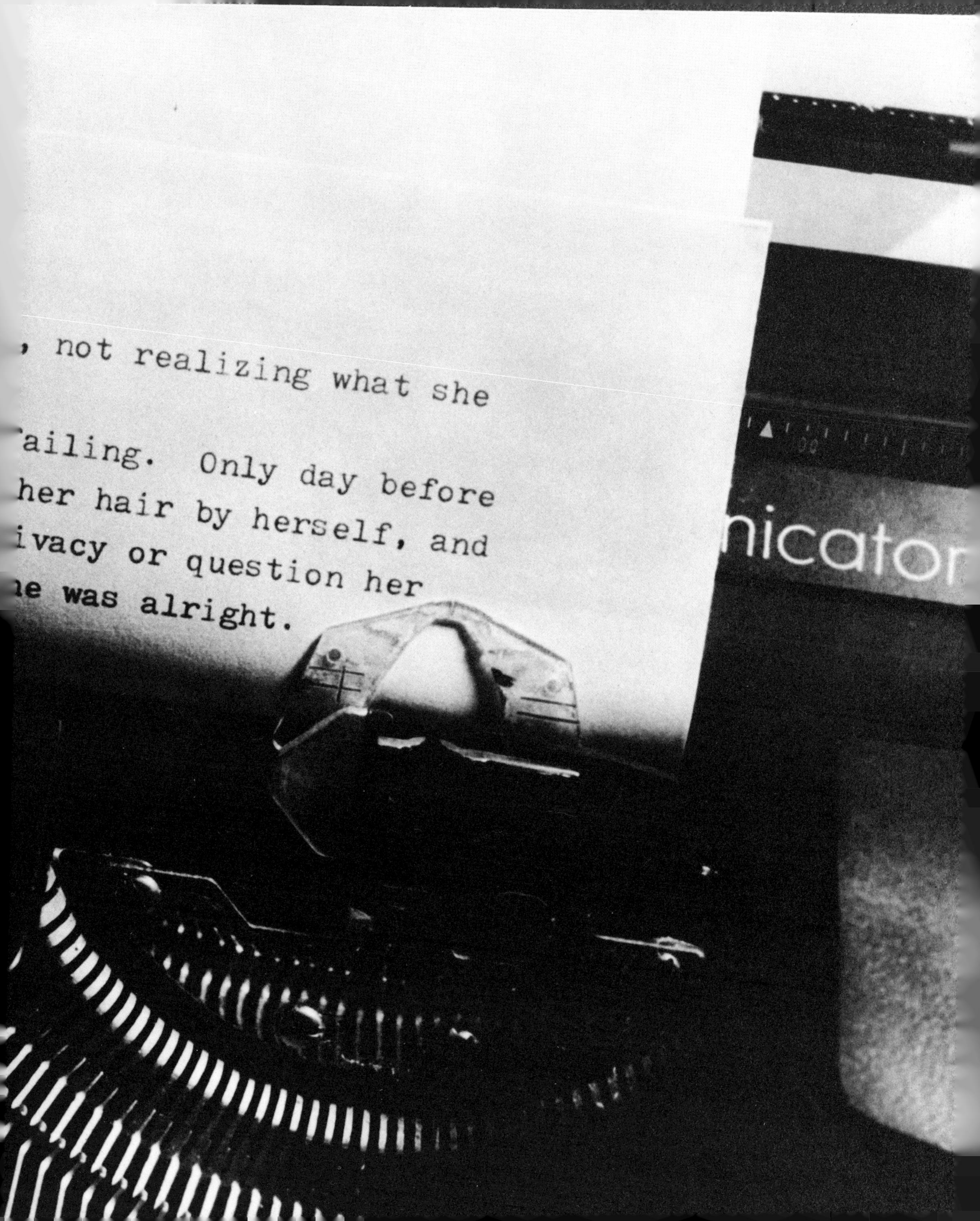
, not realizing what she
ailing. Only day before
her hair by herself, and
ivacy or question her
e was alright.
nicator

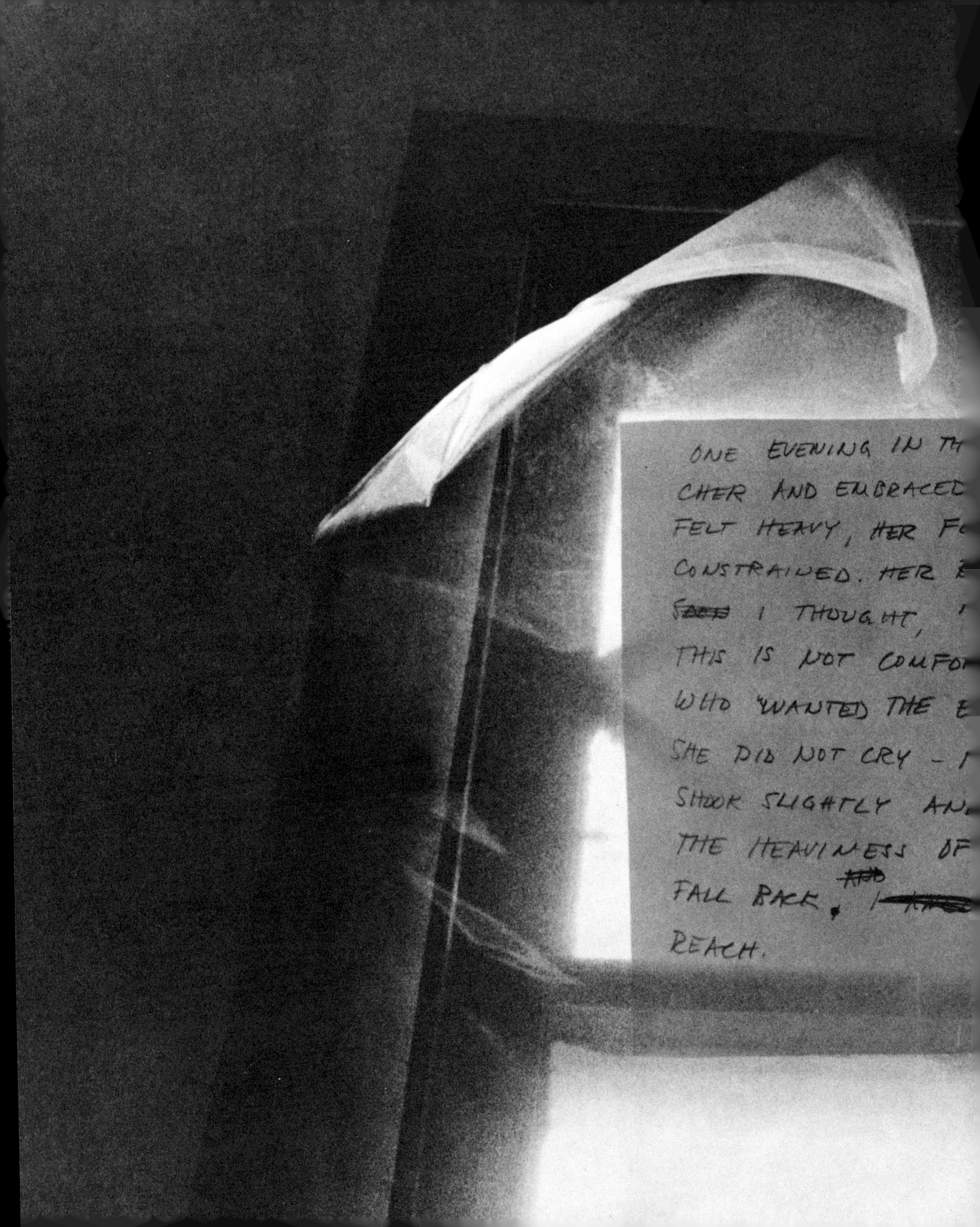
ONE EVENING IN
CHER AND
FELT HEAVY, HER
CONSTRAINED. HER
I THOUGHT,
THIS IS NOT
WHO WANTED THE
SHE DID NOT CRY -
SHOOK SLIGHTLY
THE HEAVINESS OF
FALL BACK.
REACH.

IDDLE OF THE WEEK I HELD
ER, HELD HER BODY CLOSE. SHE
TOO SOLID, HER MOVEMENTS
HAD LOST ALL RESILIENCY.
E WANTS TO LIE DOWN,
BLE FOR HER." IT WAS I
RACE. SHE DID NOT RESPOND.
FLOW OF TEARS - BUT
HIMPERED. I FELT
IC BODY, ITS TENDENCY TO
HE WAS FAR BEYOND MY

I thought it wrong to intrude o
independence by checking to mak
I spent the night with Cher in
movements sudden and unpredicta
out of bed. She rubbed her sca
hand, groaning constantly and s
Nothing I did seemed to help.
with her. Melissa woke at abou
Lou went in to calm Melissa. I
for a long time. At about 5:30

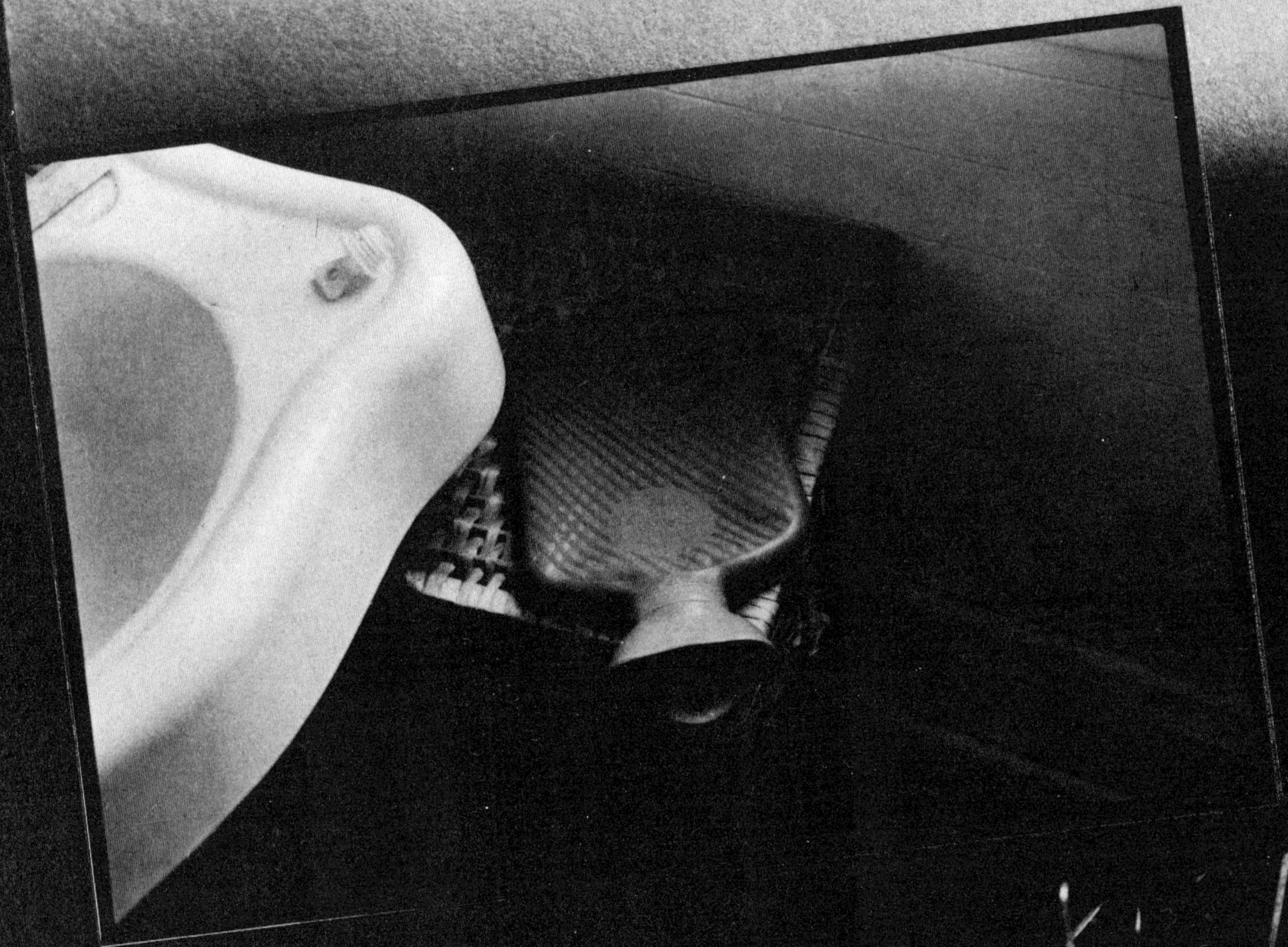

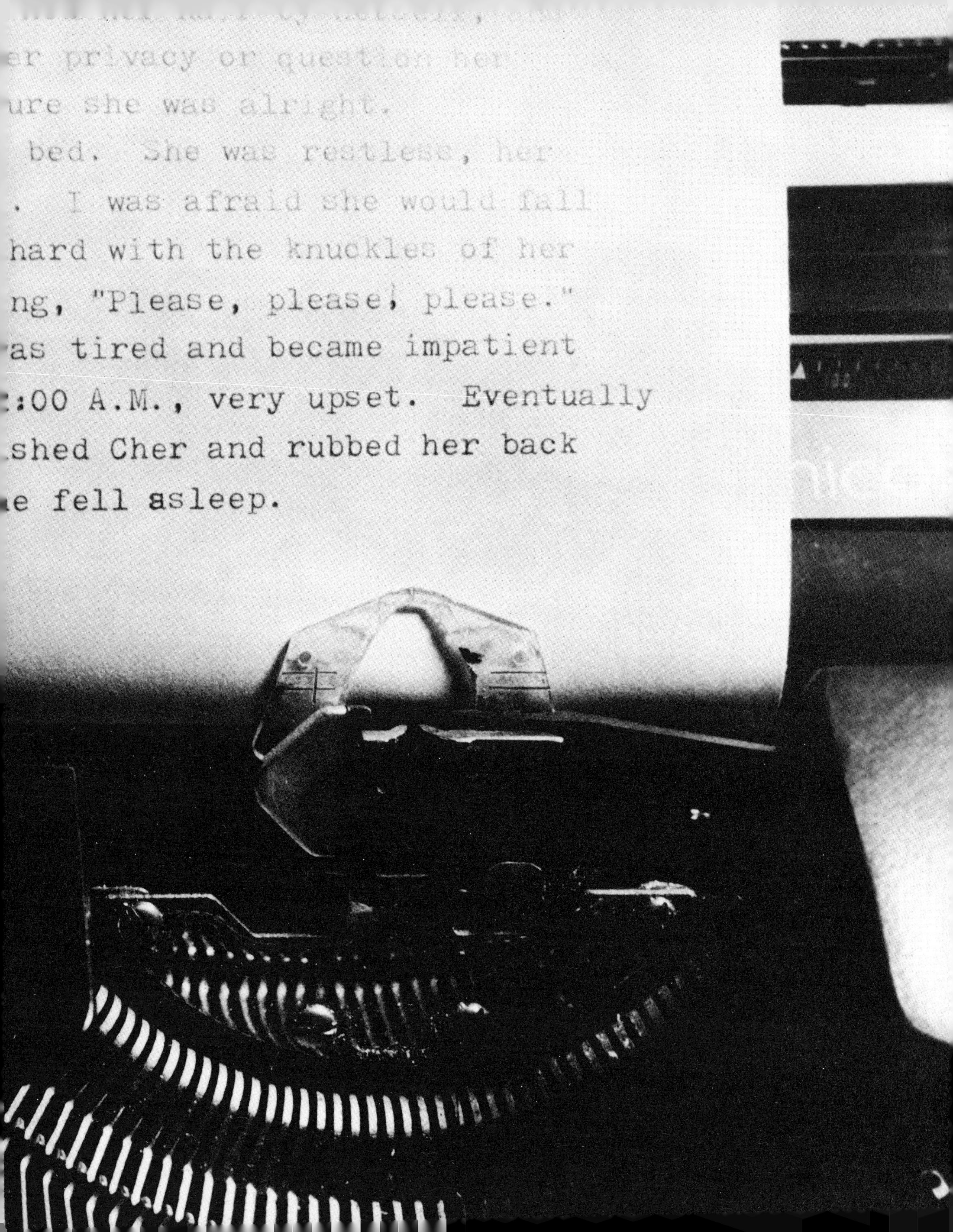
er privacy or question her
ure she was alright.
bed. She was restless, her
. I was afraid she would fall
hard with the knuckles of her
ng, "Please, please! please."
as tired and became impatient
:00 A.M., very upset. Eventually
shed Cher and rubbed her back
e fell asleep.

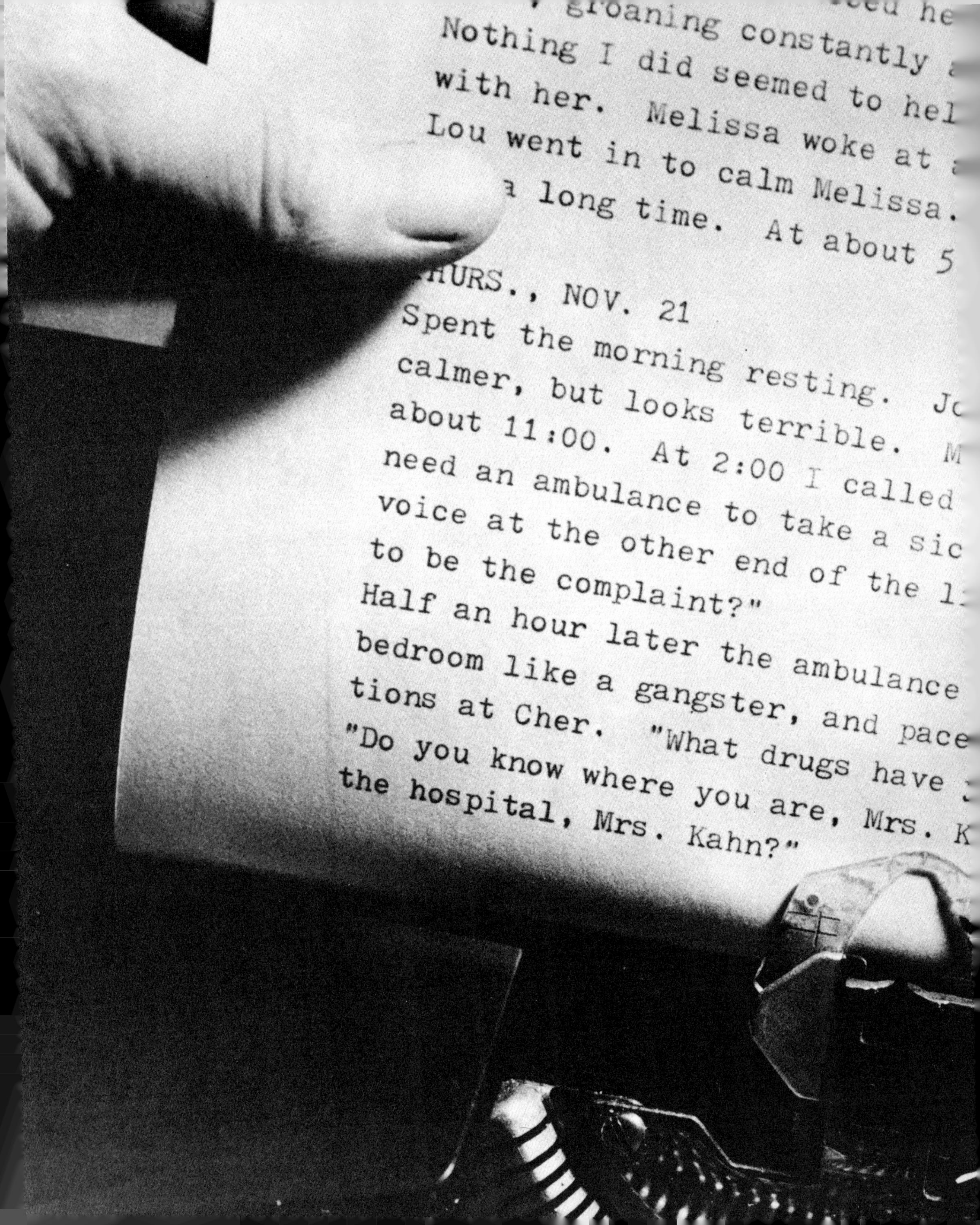
groaning constantly
Nothing I did seemed to hel
with her. Melissa woke at
Lou went in to calm Melissa.
a long time. At about 5
HURS., NOV. 21
Spent the morning resting.
calmer, but looks terrible.
about 11:00. At 2:00 I called
need an ambulance to take a sic
voice at the other end of the
to be the complaint?"
Half an hour later the ambulance
bedroom like a gangster, and pace
tions at Cher. "What drugs have
"Do you know where you are, Mrs.
the hospital, Mrs. Kahn?"

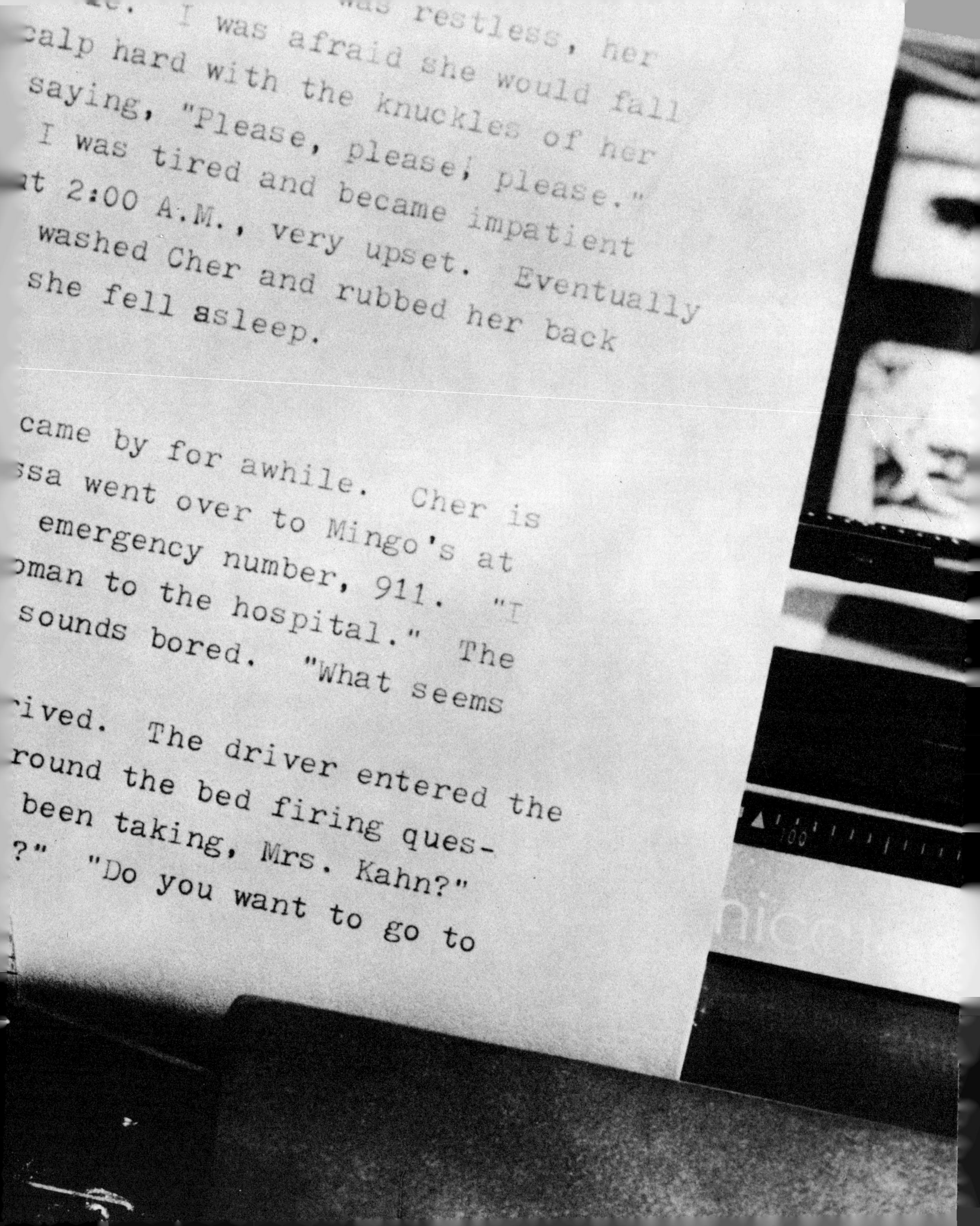
was restless, her
I was afraid she would fall
calp hard with the knuckles of her
saying, "Please, please, please."
I was tired and became impatient
at 2:00 A.M., very upset. Eventually
washed Cher and rubbed her back
she fell asleep.
came by for awhile. Cher is
ssa went over to Mingo's at
emergency number, 911. "I
oman to the hospital." The
sounds bored. "What seems
rived. The driver entered the
round the bed firing ques-
been taking, Mrs. Kahn?"
?" "Do you want to go to

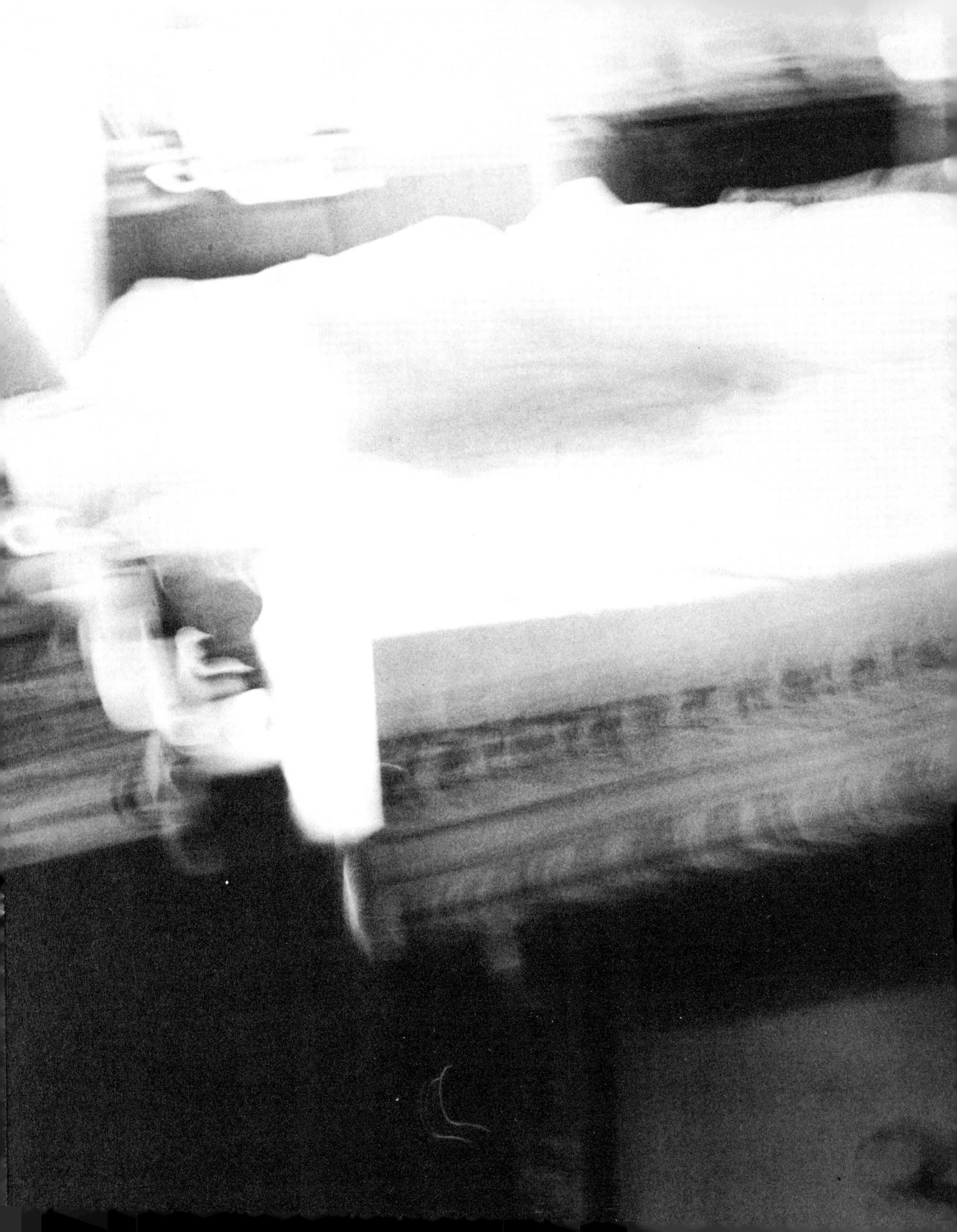

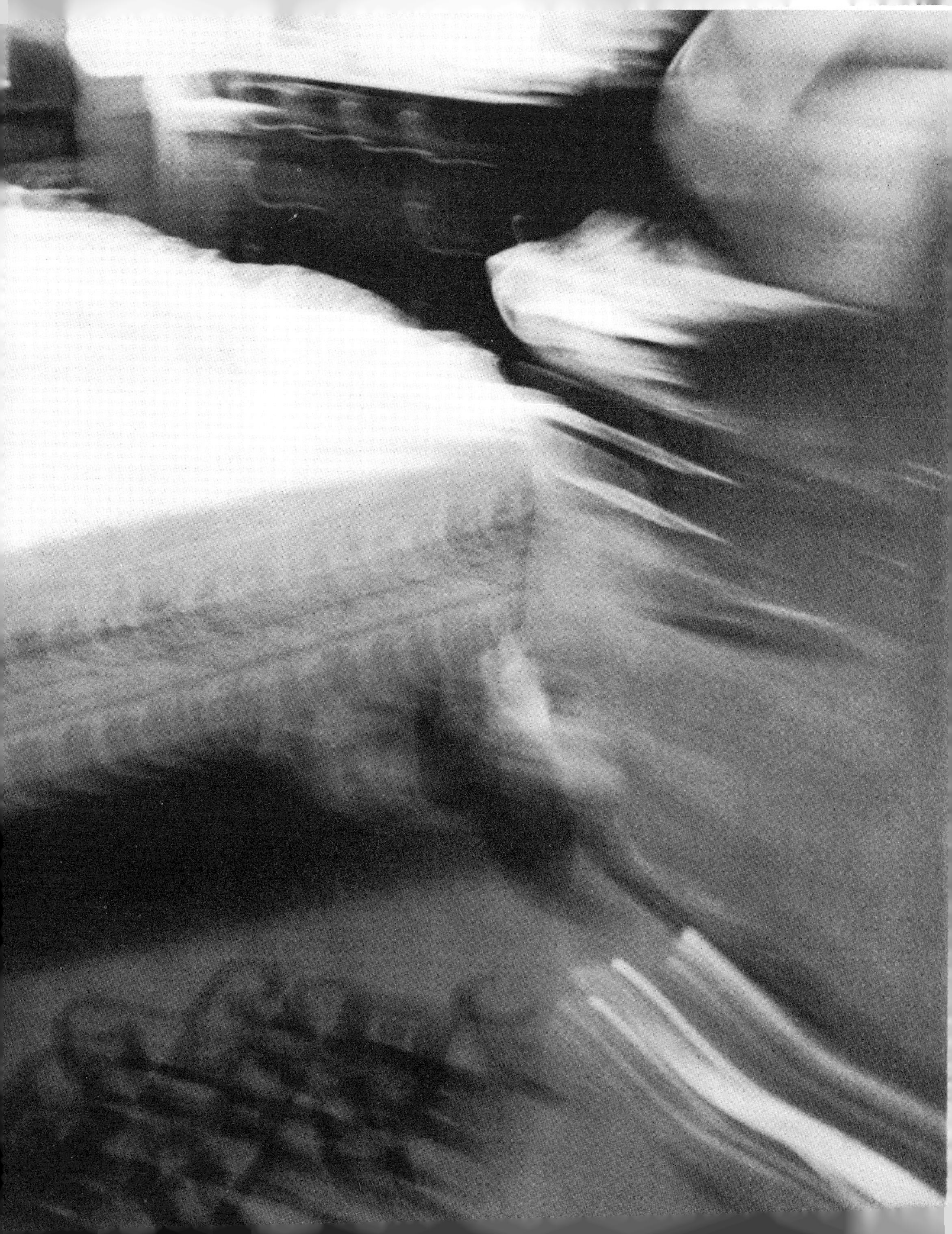

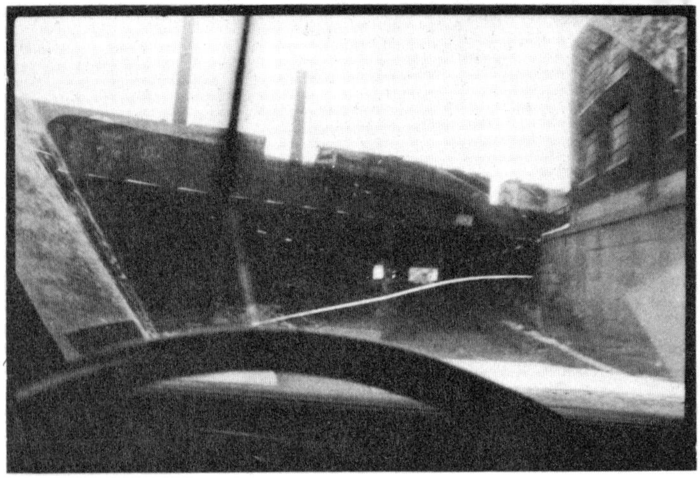
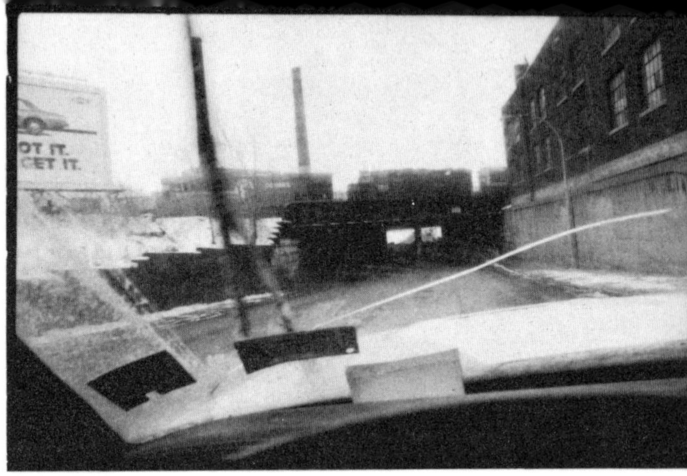
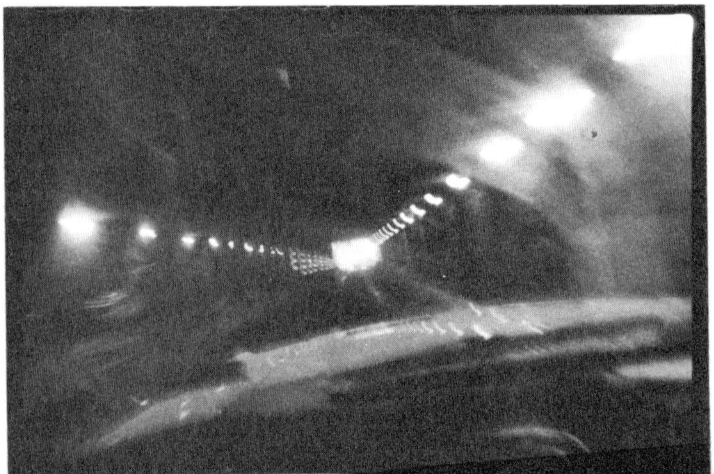
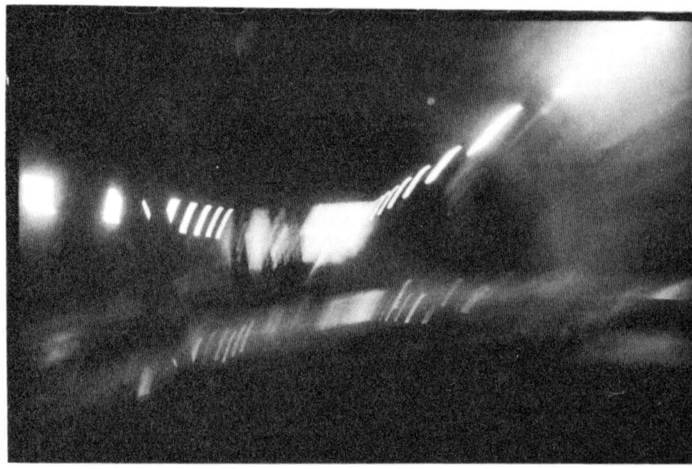
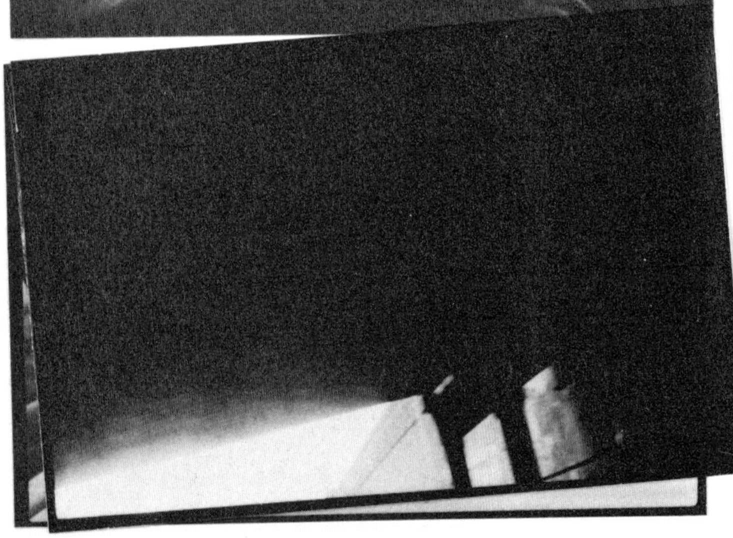
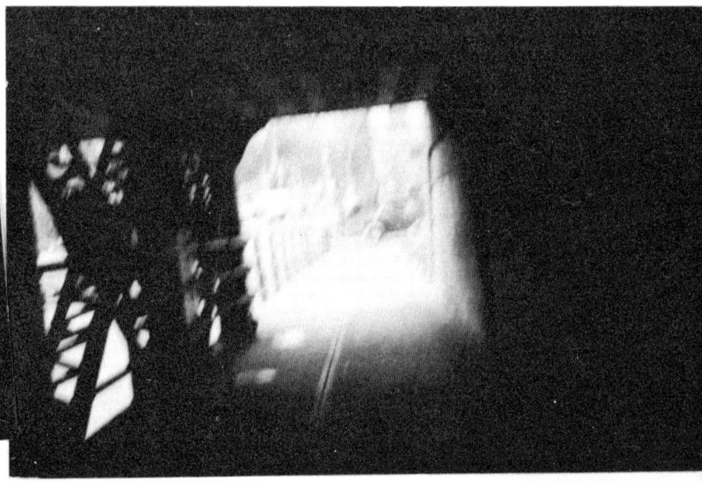

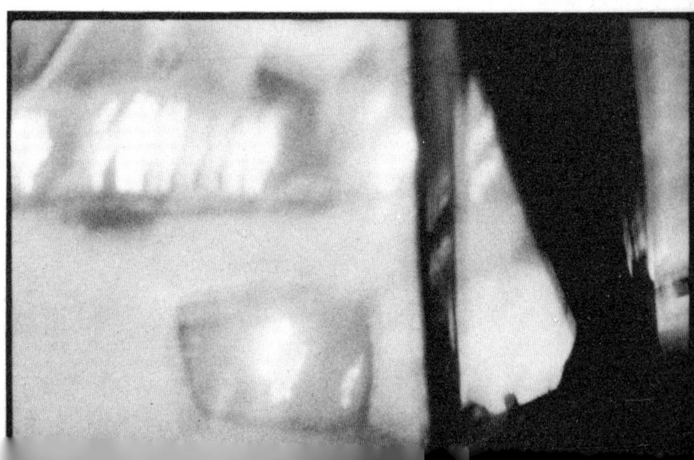

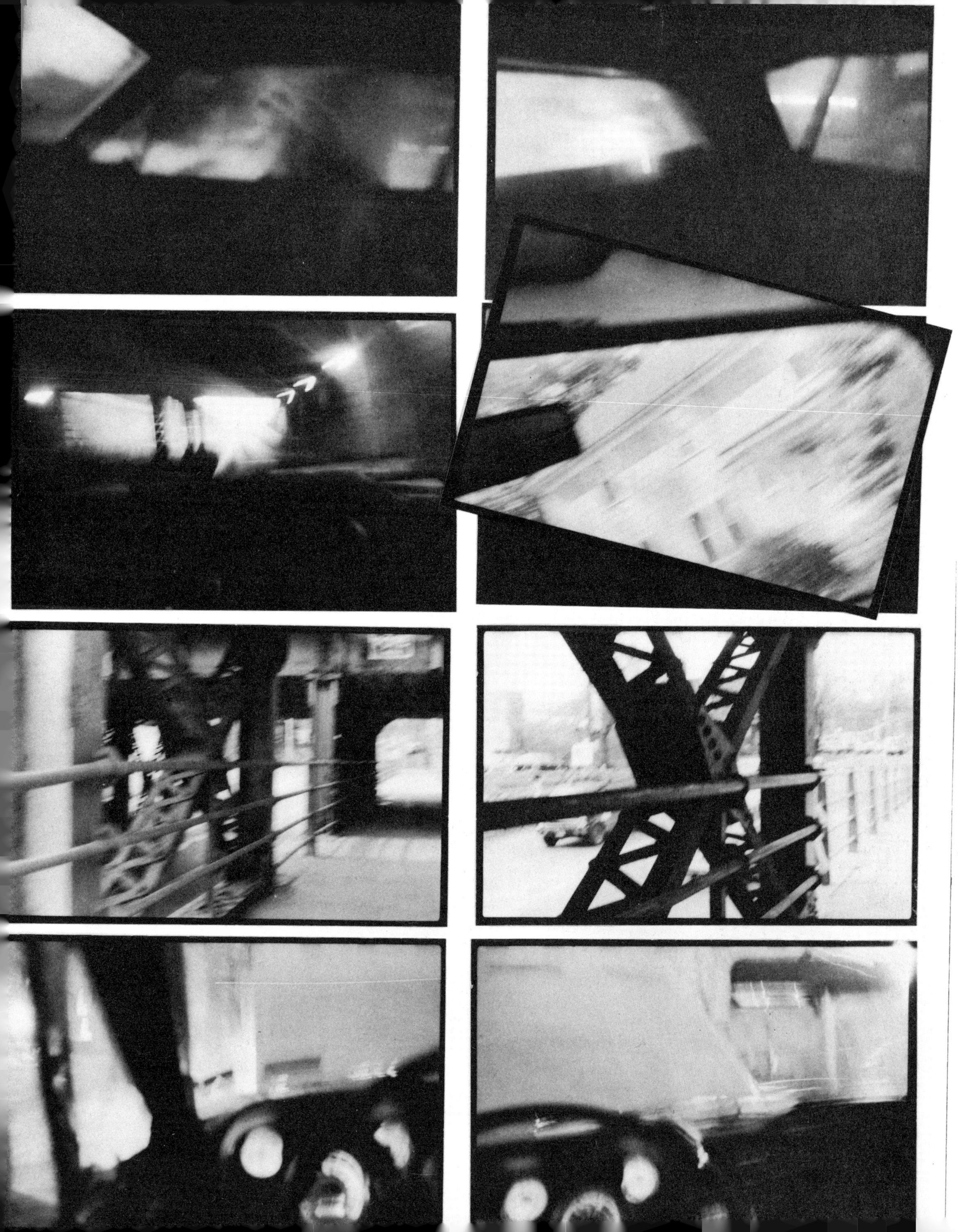

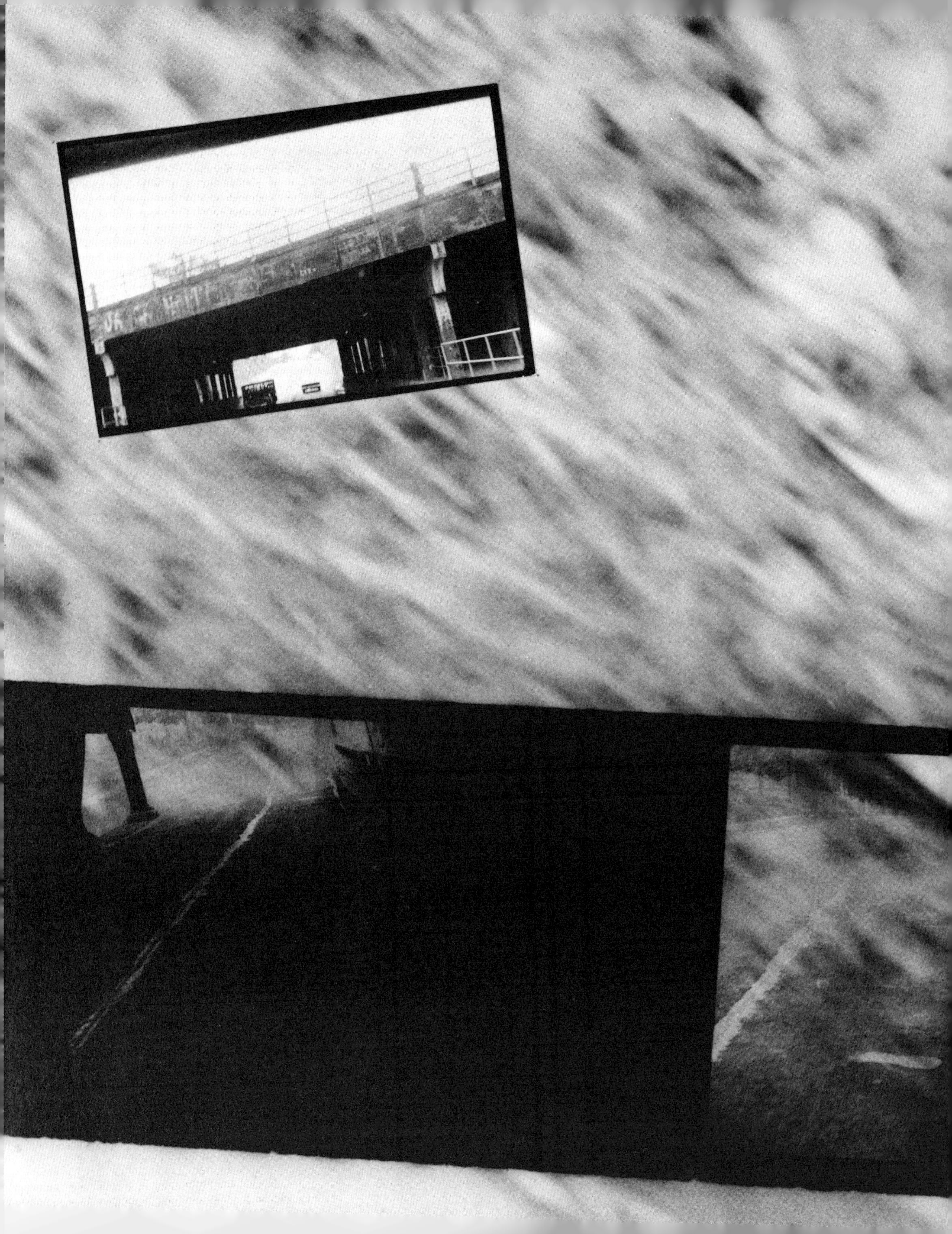

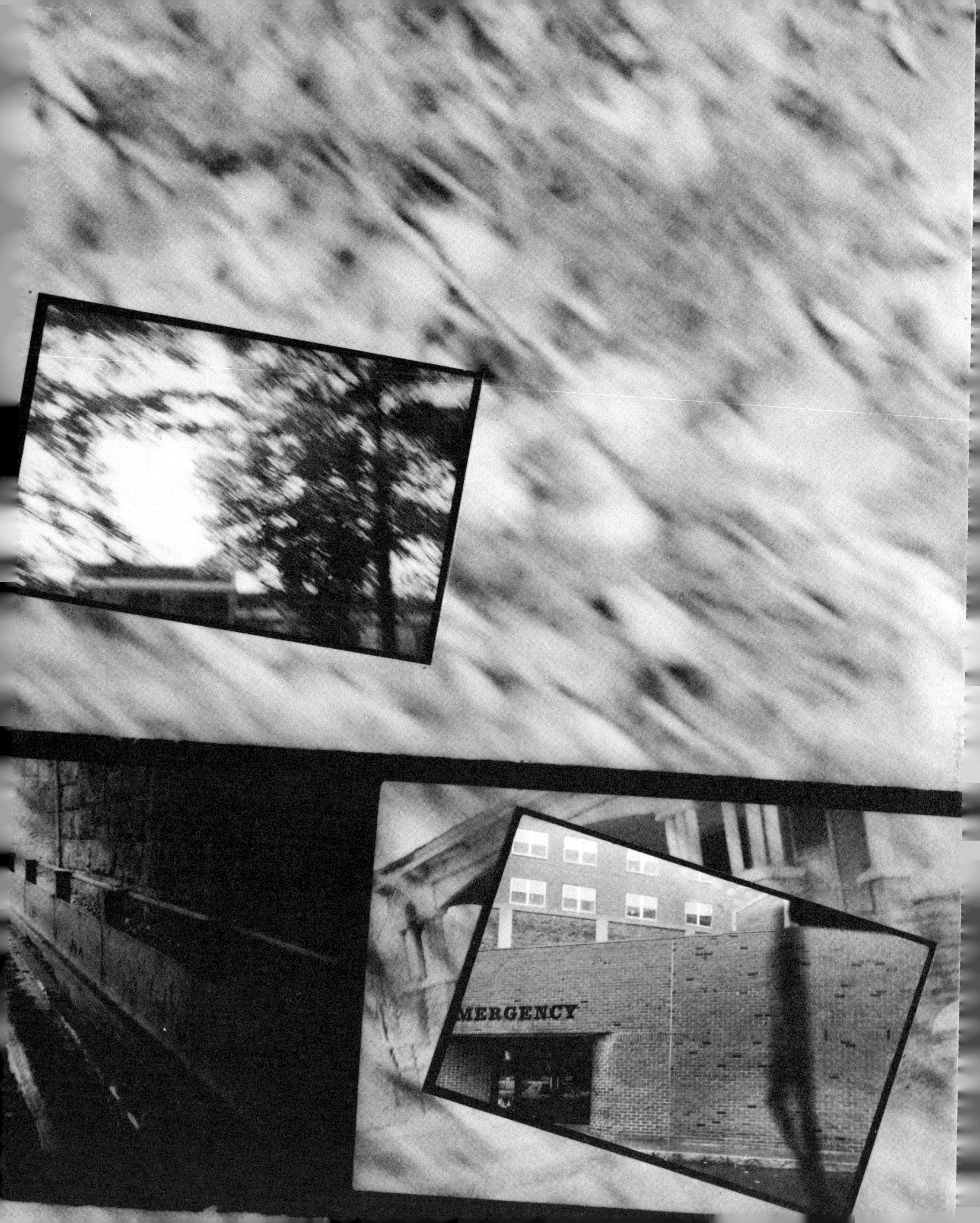
MERGENCY

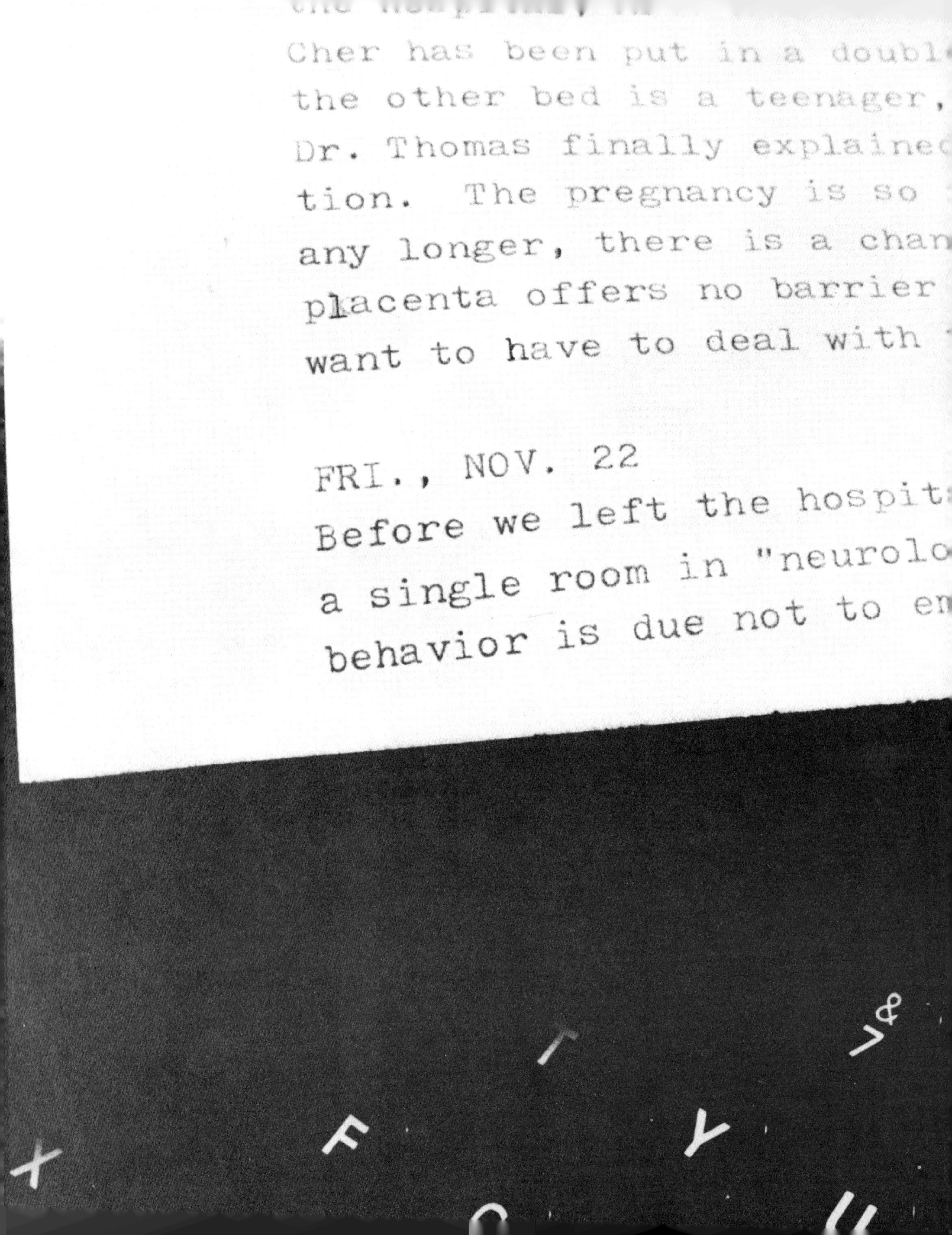
Cher has been put in a
the other bed is a teenager,
Dr. Thomas finally
tion. The pregnancy is so
any longer, there is a
placenta offers no barrier
want to have to deal with
FRI., NOV. 22
Before we left the
a single room in
behavior is due not to

oom in the OB ward. Th

ccompanied by her mother.

o me why Cher must have this abor-

advanced now that if they wait

the foetus may be born alive. The

the cancer. The doctors do not

t situation.

last night they had moved Cher to

". It is now recognized that her

ional hysteria or depression, but

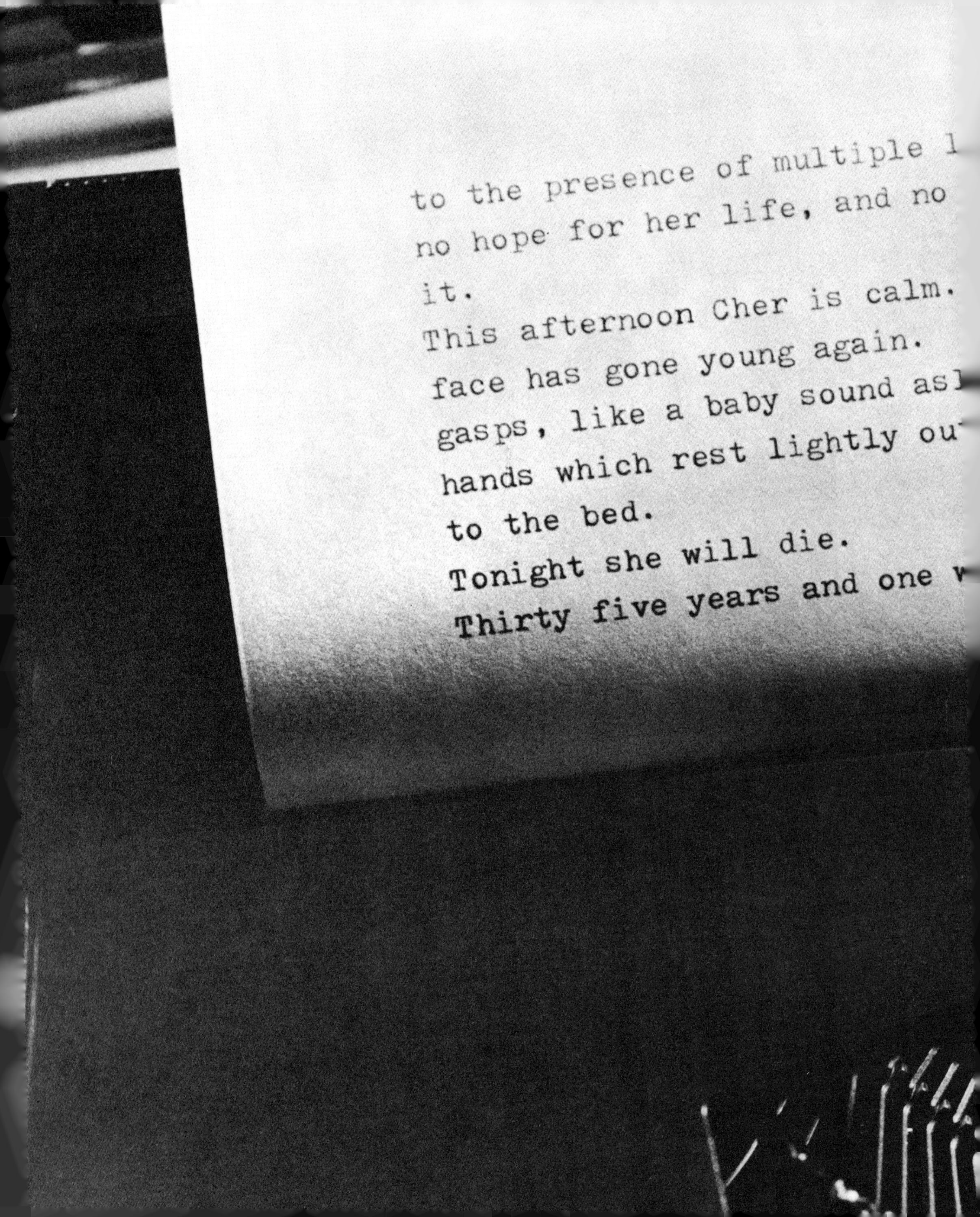
to the presence of multiple
no hope for her life, and no
it.
This afternoon Cher is calm.
face has gone young again.
gasps, like a baby sound
hands which rest lightly
to the bed.
Tonight she will die.
Thirty five years and one

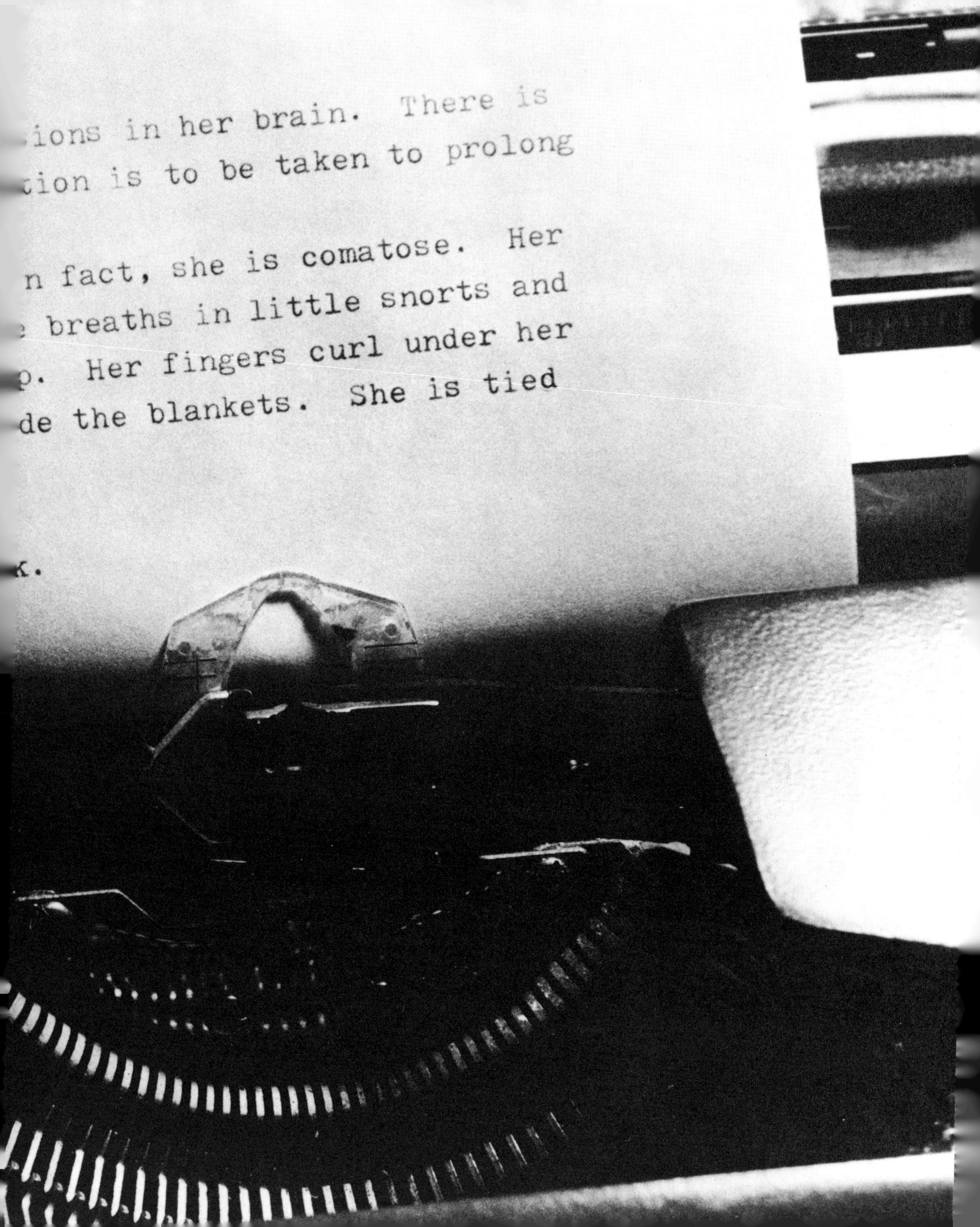
ions in her brain. There is
ion is to be taken to prolong
n fact, she is comatose. Her
breaths in little snorts and
Her fingers curl under her
de the blankets. She is tied

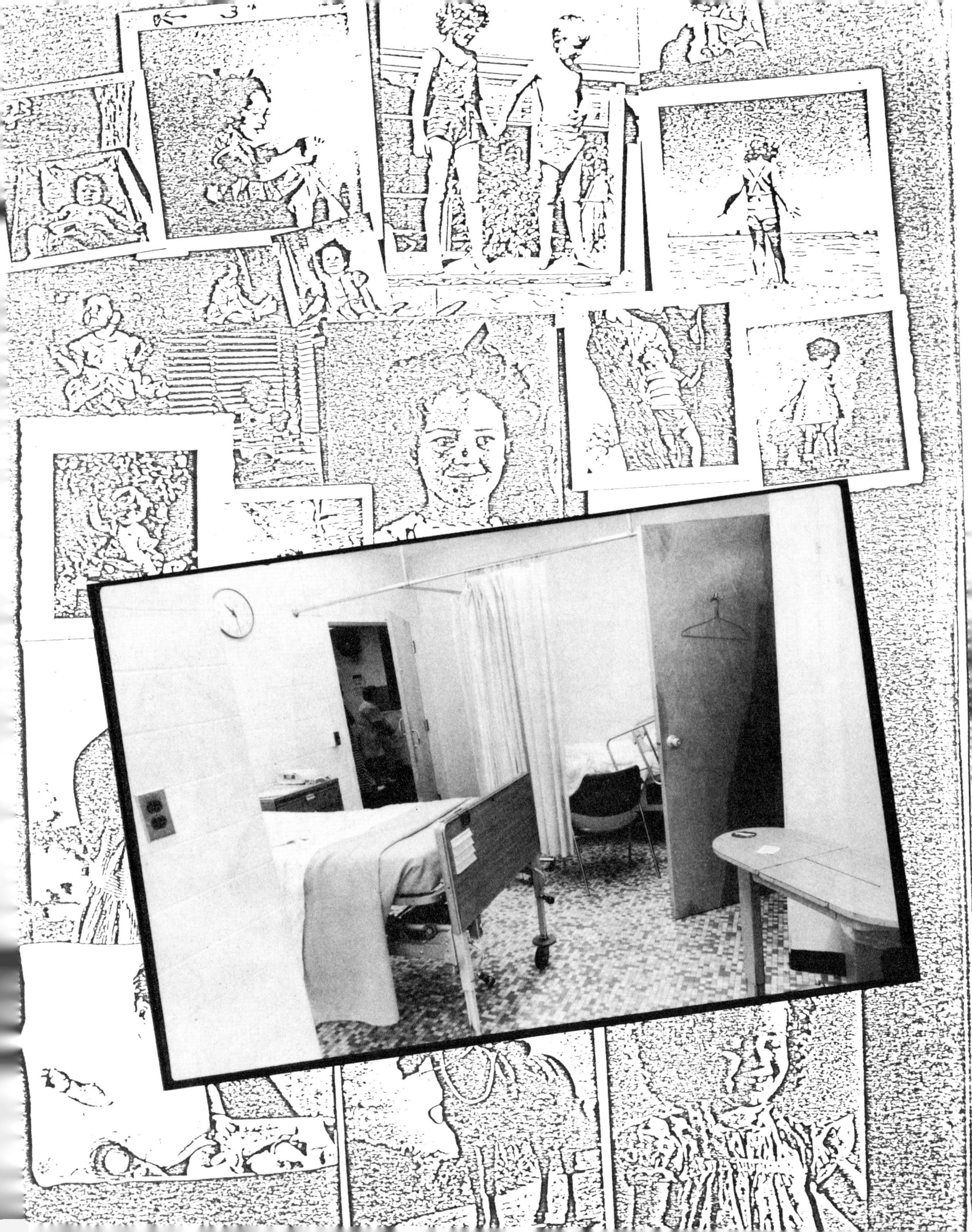

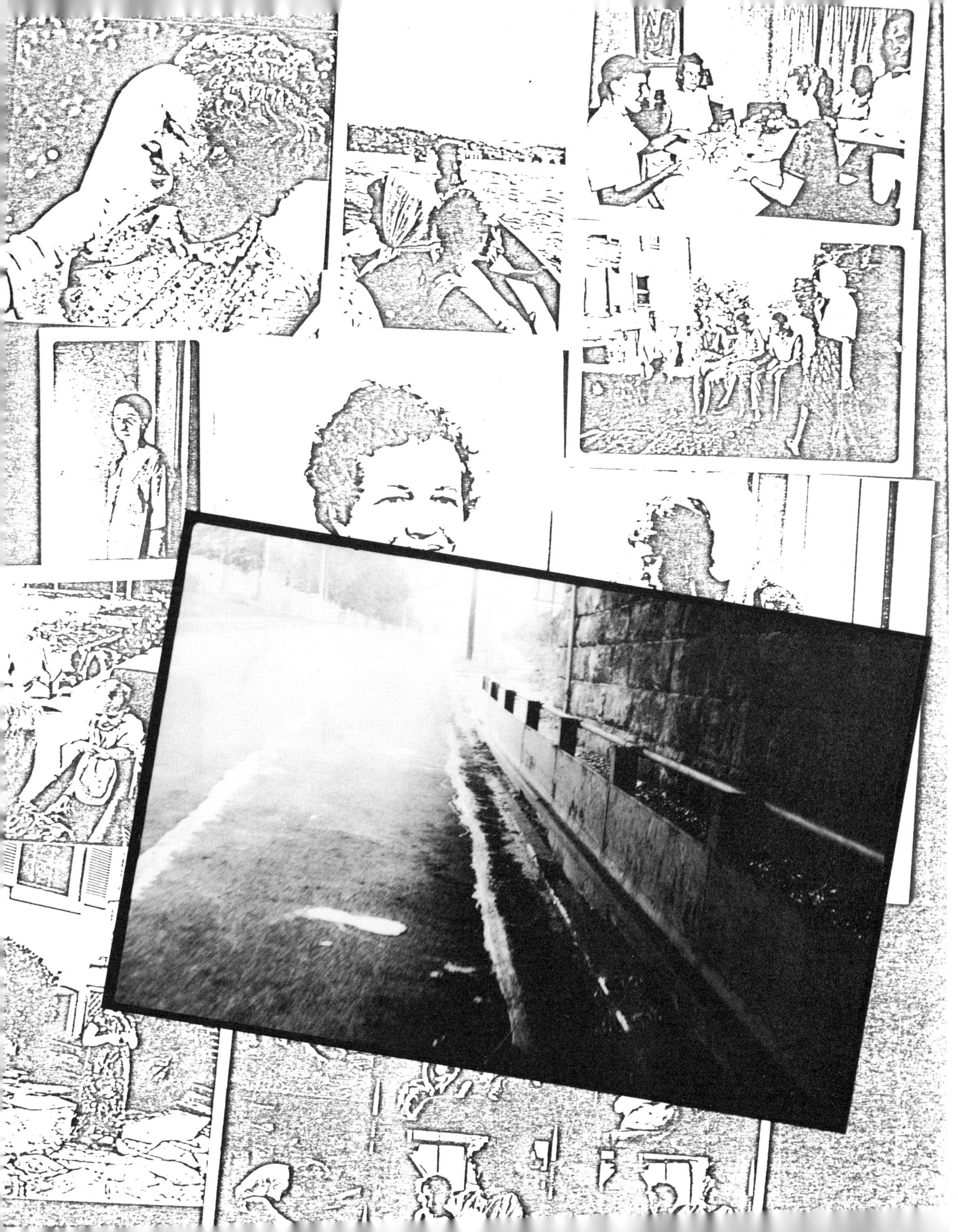

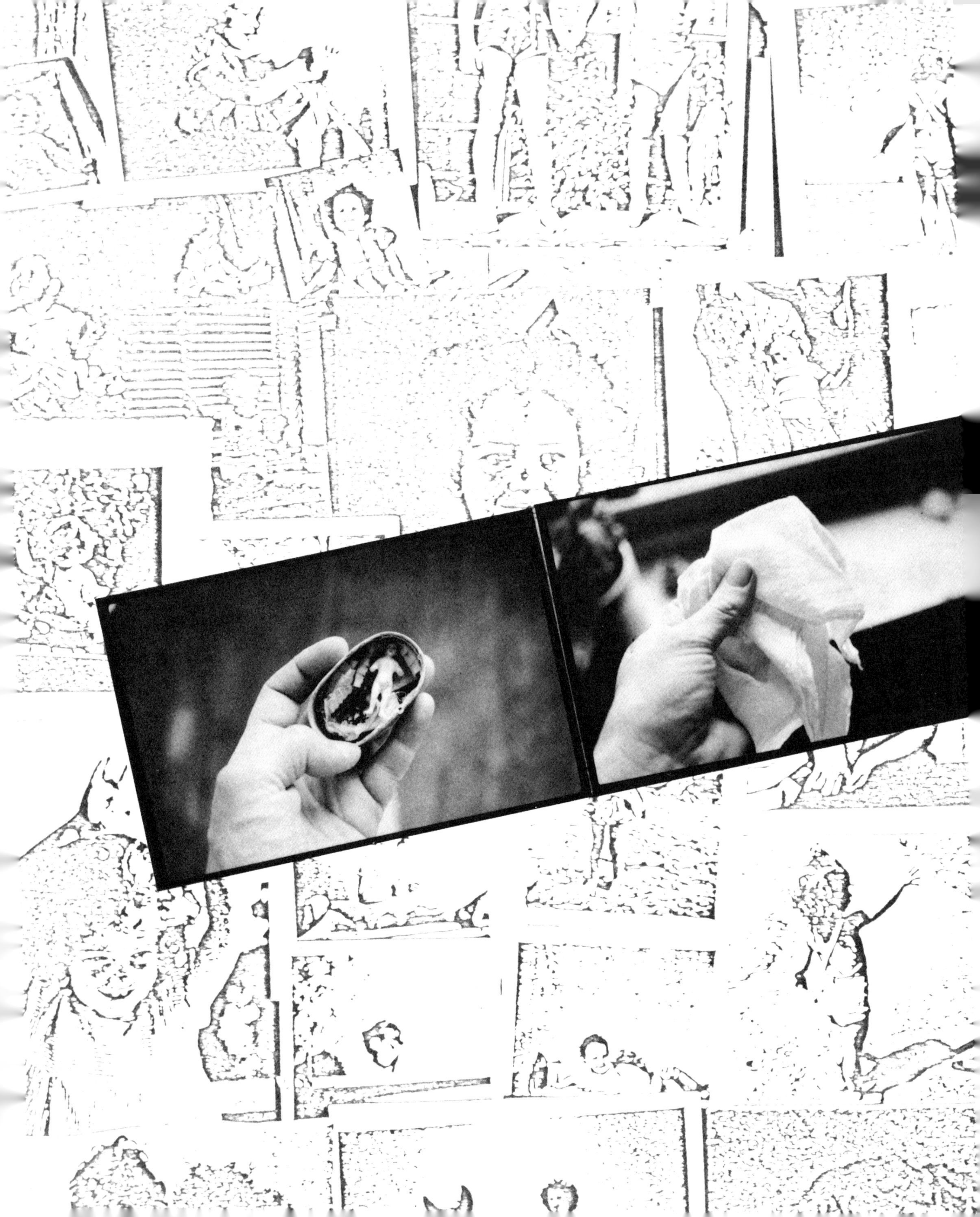

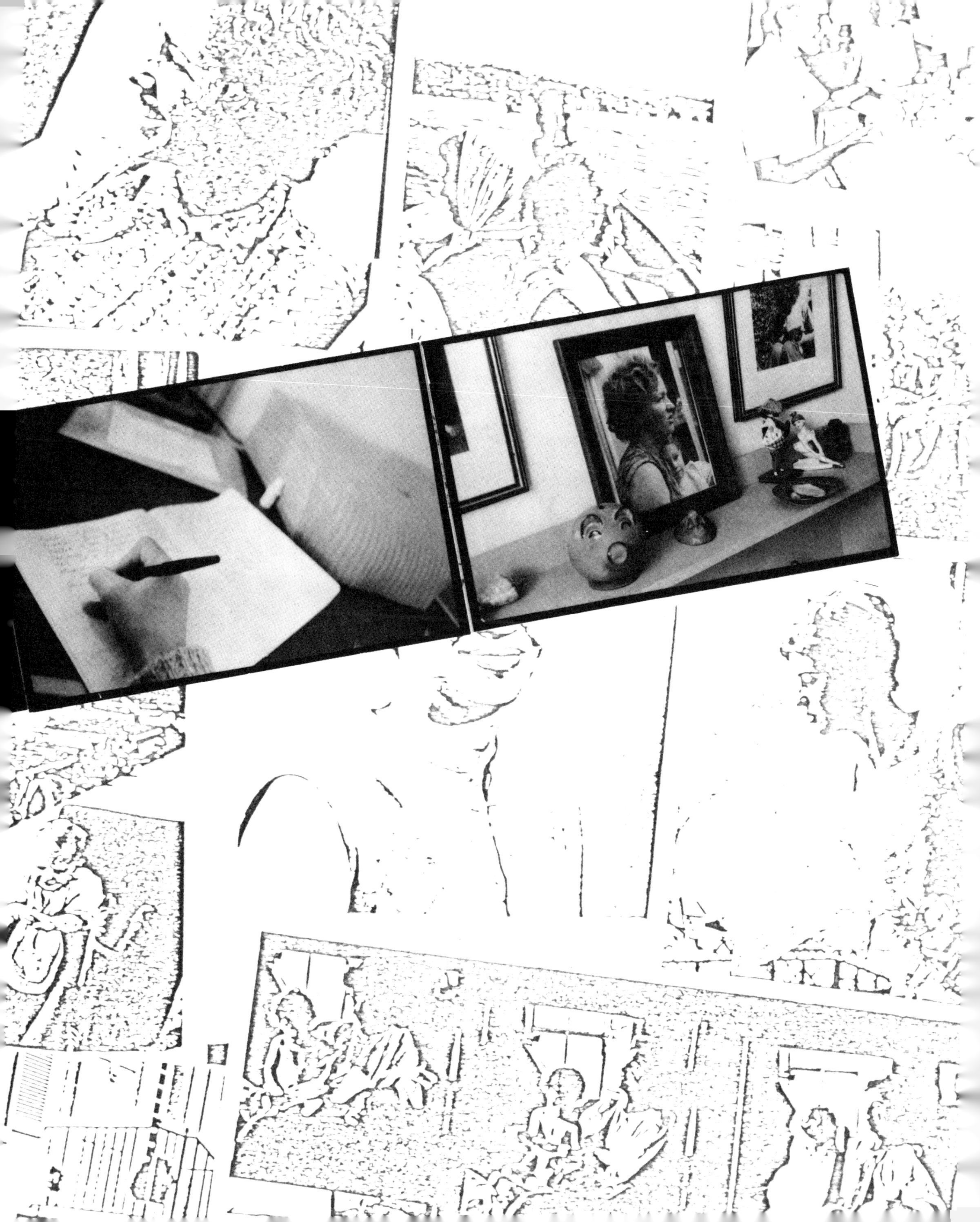

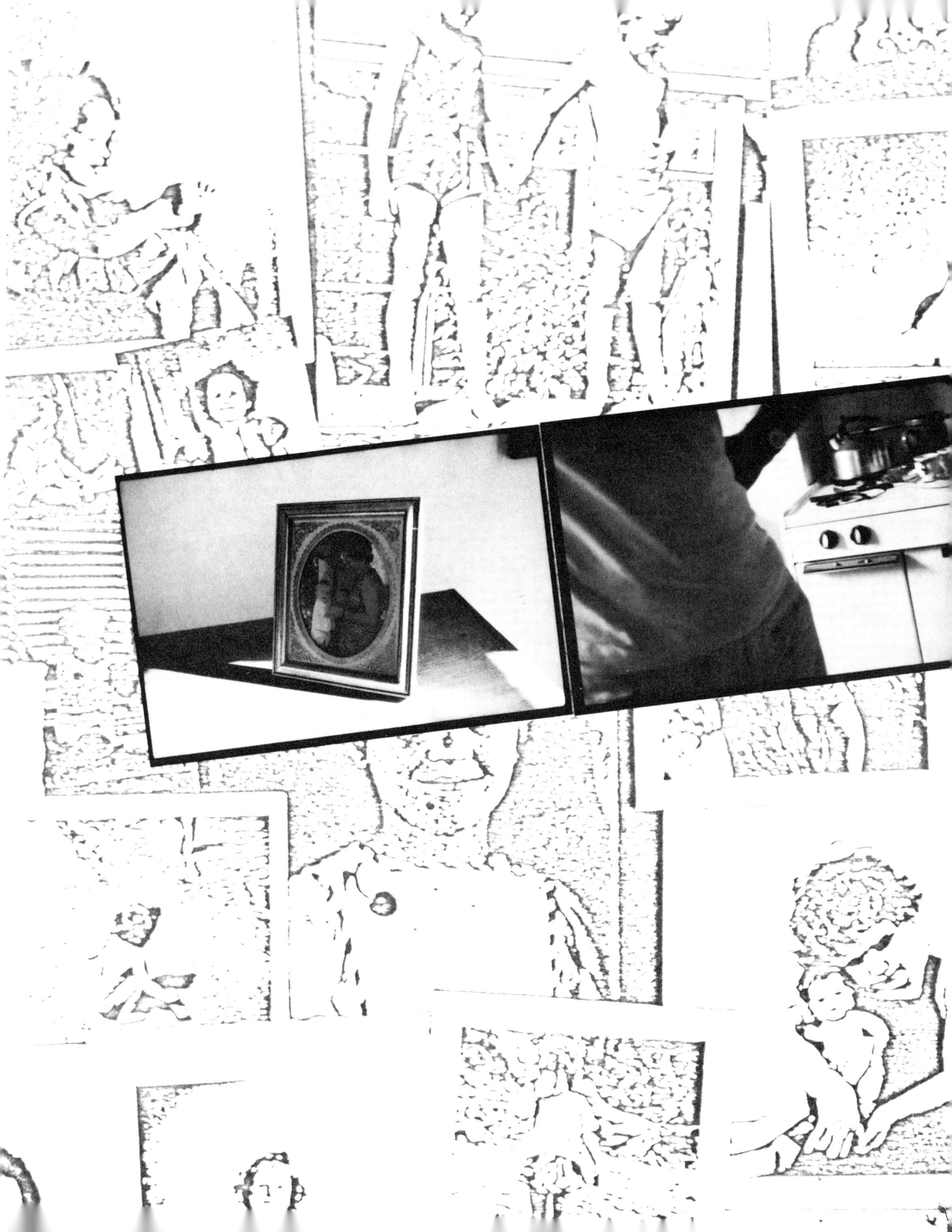

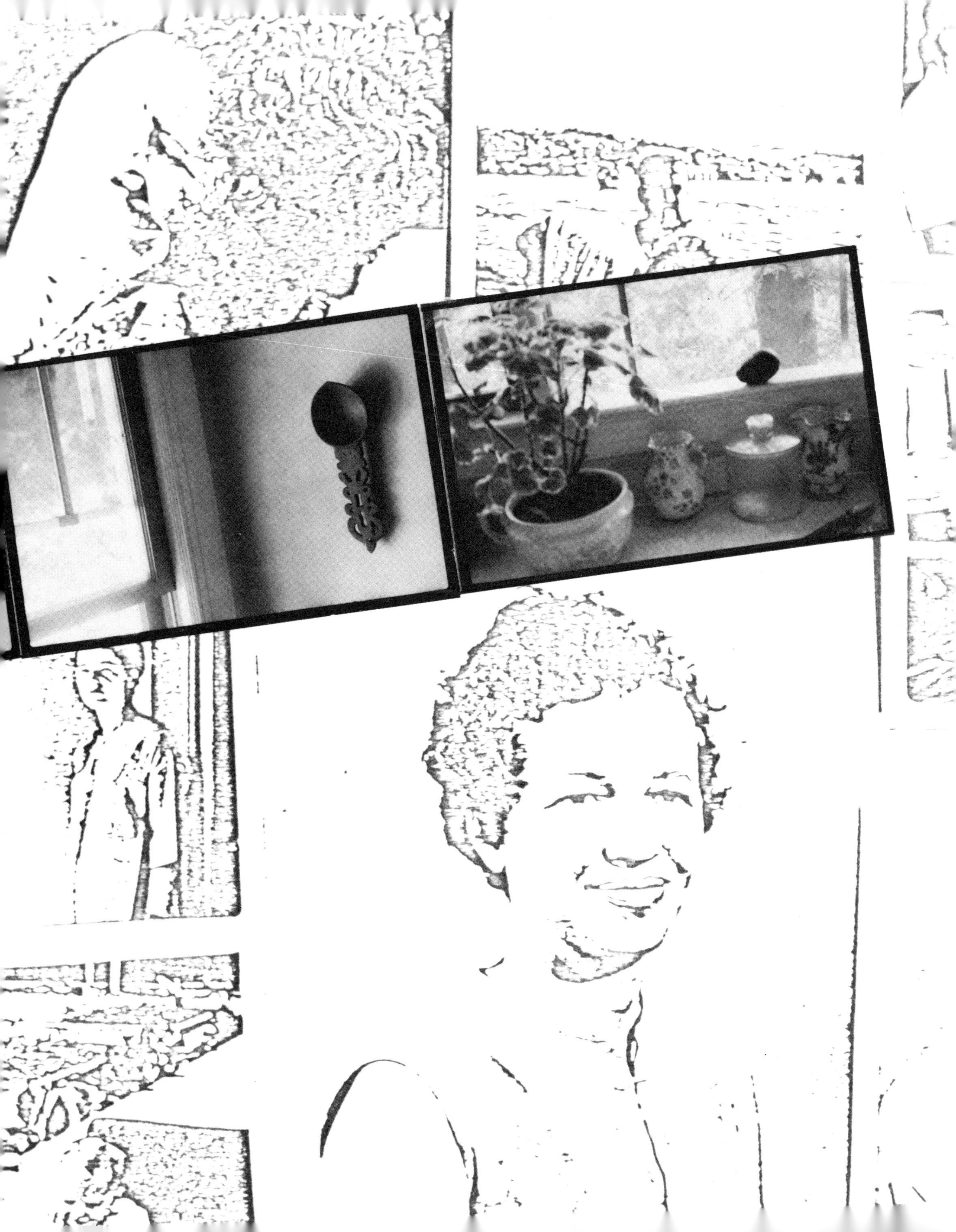

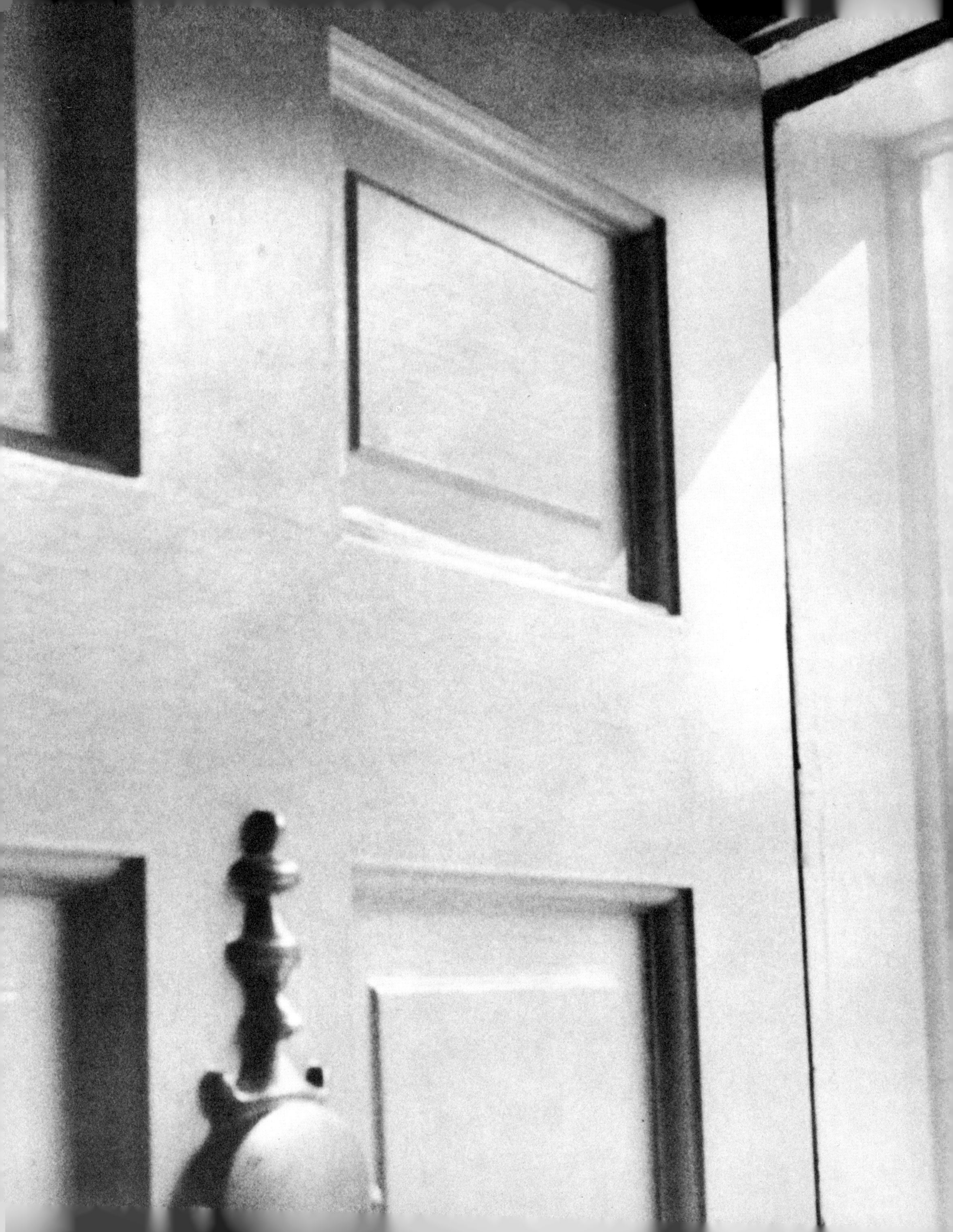

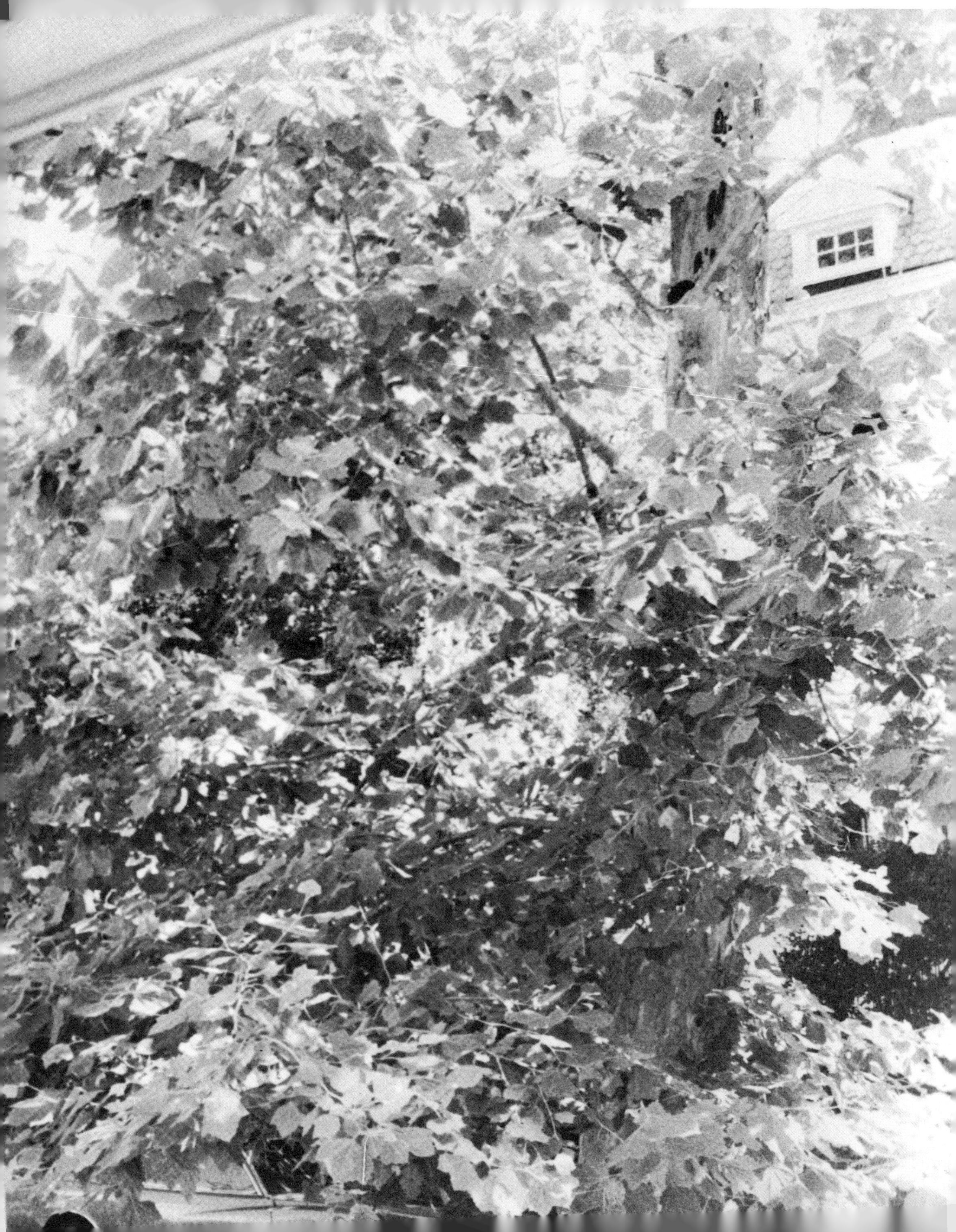

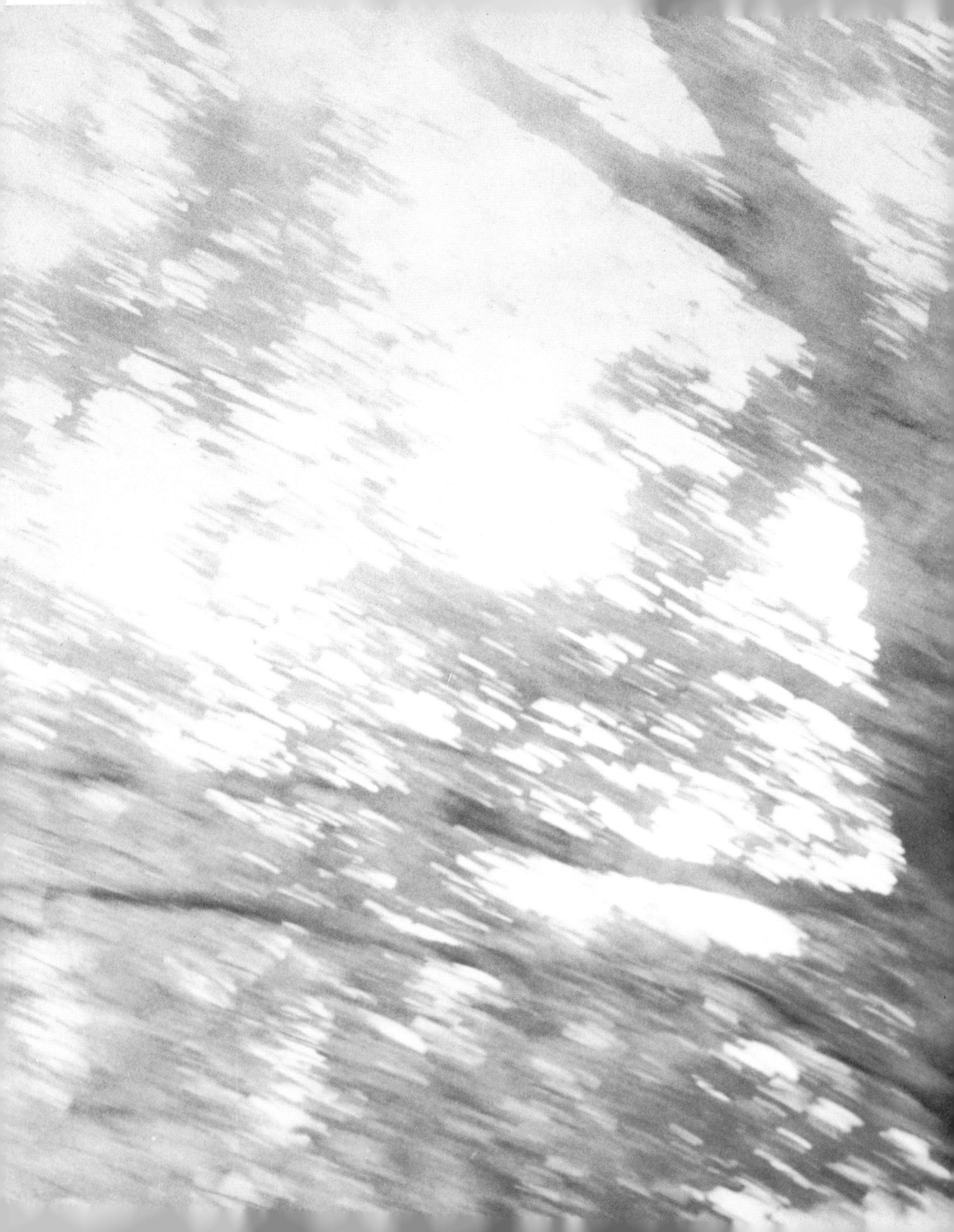